# FOOD AND COOKERY
# FOR THE SICK
### AND
# CONVALESCENT

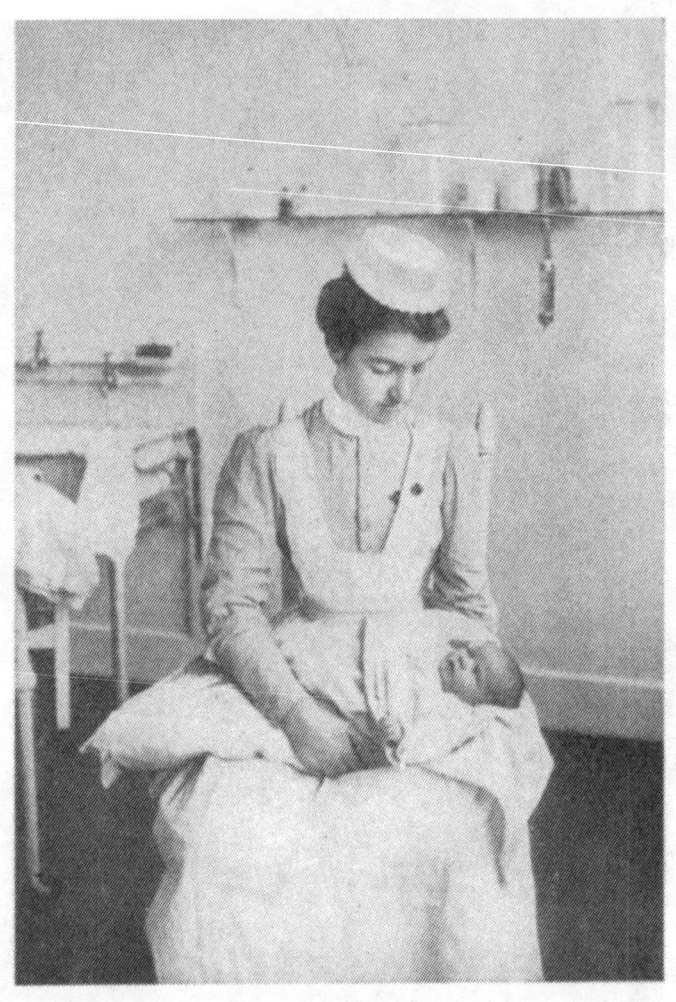

A HEALTHY FEMALE INFANT

Weight at Birth: Seven and one-half pounds.   Age: Nine days.

*Taken by courtesy of The Maternity Department,
Massachusetts Homœopathic Hospital, Boston.*

# FOOD AND COOKERY
# FOR THE SICK
### AND
# CONVALESCENT

BY

**FANNIE MERRITT FARMER**

PRINCIPAL OF MISS FARMER'S SCHOOL OF COOKERY

AND AUTHOR OF

"THE BOSTON COOKING-SCHOOL COOK BOOK" AND

"CHAFING-DISH POSSIBILITIES"

**Creative Cookbooks**
**Monterey, California**

Food and Cookery for the Sick and Convalescent

by
Fannie Merrditt Farmer

ISBN: 1-58963-375-X

Copyright © 2001 by Fredonia Books

Reprinted from the 1911 edition

Creative Cookbooks
An Imprint of Fredonia Books
Monterey, California
http://www.creativecookbooks.com

All rights reserved, including the right to reproduce this book, or portions thereof, in any form.

In order to make original editions of historical works available to scholars at an economical price, this facsimile of the original edition of 1911 is reproduced from the best available copy and has been digitally enhanced to improve legibility, but the text remains unaltered to retain historical authenticity.

TO

## MY MOTHER

WHOSE DEVOTION TO DUTY HAS INSPIRED ME TO
MY BEST WORK

𝔗𝔥𝔦𝔰 𝔅𝔬𝔬𝔨 𝔦𝔰 𝔏𝔬𝔳𝔦𝔫𝔤𝔩𝔶 𝔇𝔢𝔡𝔦𝔠𝔞𝔱𝔢𝔡

*"Invalid Cookery should form the basis of every trained nurse's education."*

*A good sick cook will save the digestion half its work.*
          FLORENCE NIGHTINGALE

*The careful preparation of food is now recognized to be of vital importance to an invalid, and a valuable assistance, in many cases, to the physician, in hastening the recovery of a patient.*
          HELENA V. SACHSE

# PREFACE.

"*Food is the only source of human power to work or to think.*"

THIS work is designed to meet the demands made upon me by the numberless classes of trained nurses whom it has been my pleasure and privilege to instruct during my thirteen years of service as a teacher of cookery.

It is earnestly hoped that, besides meeting this long felt need, it will do a still broader work in thousands of homes throughout the land, where it will be of inestimable help to the mothers upon whom so much of the welfare of the family depends.

The opening chapters are equally valuable to those who care for the sick and those who see in correct feeding the way of preventing much of the illness about us.

Emphasis has been laid on the importance of diet from infancy to old age. The classification, composition, nutritive value, and digestibility of foods have been carefully considered with the same constant purpose of being a help to those who arrange dietaries. The chapter on infant feeding is an authoritative guide to aid in the development of the baby, while child feeding is considered with like care. Considerable matter has been introduced with reference to diet in various diseases, and the recipes for the diebetic have involved much thought and labor.

The hundreds of thoroughly tested recipes cover the whole range of the subject of cookery for the sick and convalescent. They are, for the most part, individual, thus requiring but a minimum of time for their preparation, while many have their caloric value given.

I wish to express my sincere thanks for the sympathy, encouragement, and help I have received from pupils, superintendents of nurses, professors, and physicians, which have made this work possible.

F. M. F.

# TABLE OF CONTENTS.

| Chapter | | Page |
|---|---|---|
| I. | Food and its Relation to the Body | 1 |
| II. | Estimates of Food Values | 7 |
| III. | Digestion | 12 |
| IV. | Food and Health vs. Drugs and Disease | 18 |
| V. | Infant Feeding | 21 |
| VI. | Child Feeding | 30 |
| VII. | Food for the Sick | 36 |
| VIII. | Cookery for the Sick | 41 |
| IX. | Water | 46 |
| X. | Milk | 50 |
| XI. | Alcohol | 58 |
| XII. | Beverages | 62 |
| XIII. | Gruels, Beef Extracts, and Beef Teas | 82 |
| XIV. | Bread | 88 |
| XV. | Breakfast Cereals | 100 |
| XVI. | Eggs | 106 |
| XVII. | Soups, Broths, and Stews | 118 |
| XVIII. | Fish | 125 |
| XIX. | Meat | 134 |
| XX. | Vegetables | 151 |
| XXI. | Potatoes | 159 |
| XXII. | Salads and Sandwiches | 163 |

## TABLE OF CONTENTS.

| Chapter | | Page |
|---|---|---|
| XXIII. | Hot Puddings and Pudding Sauces | 172 |
| XXIV. | Jellies | 179 |
| XXV. | Cold Desserts | 187 |
| XXVI. | Frozen Desserts | 196 |
| XXVII. | Fruits and how to Serve them | 203 |
| XXVIII. | Wafers and Cakes | 211 |
| XXIX. | Diabetes | 217 |
| XXX. | Diet in Special Diseases | 246 |

Indexes:
    Technical and Descriptive . . . . . . . . 265
    Recipes . . . . . . . . . . . . . . . 277

# LIST OF ILLUSTRATIONS.

| | |
|---|---:|
| A Healthy Female Infant | *Frontispiece* |
| | **FACING PAGE** |
| Infant's Water-Bottle, Nursing-Bottle, and Nipple | 16 |
| Breakfast Tray | 17 |
| Luncheon Trays | 32 |
| One-half pint tin Measuring Cups and Teaspoons, illustrating the Measuring of Dry Ingredients | 33 |
| Necessary Utensils for Invalid Cookery | 36 |
| Drinking Cups and Glass Drinking Tube or Siphon | 37 |
| Medicine Glass with Glass Cover and Ideal Glass | 37 |
| Currant Jelly Water | 44 |
| Bread Dough, with Suggestions for Shaping. Zwieback | 45 |
| Shirred Egg | 48 |
| Egg in a Nest | 48 |
| Utensils used in the making of Omelets | 49 |
| Broiled Fish, Garnish of Potato Border and Lemon | 64 |
| Baked Fillets of Halibut | 64 |
| Fancy Roast, garnished with Toast Points and Parsley | 65 |
| Broiled Oysters | 65 |
| Broiled Tenderloin of Beef with Beef Marrow | 80 |
| Beef cut in Strips for Scraping | 80 |
| Beef Balls | 81 |
| Beef Balls | 81 |
| Pan-broiled French Chops with Potato Balls | 96 |
| Jellied Sweetbread | 96 |

## LIST OF ILLUSTRATIONS.

|  | FACING PAGE |
|---|---|
| Creamed Chicken in Potato Border | 97 |
| Pastry Bag and Tubes | 97 |
| Boned Bird in Paper Case, ready for Broiling | 100 |
| Quail Split and ready for Broiling | 100 |
| Chicken and Rice Cutlet | 101 |
| Broiled Quail on Toast, garnished | 101 |
| Croustade of Creamed Peas | 108 |
| Egg Salad | 109 |
| Sweetbread and Celery Salad, garnished with Red and Green Pepper cut in Narrow Strips | 109 |
| Bread and Butter Sandwiches | 112 |
| Entire Wheat Bread Sandwiches | 112 |
| Dinner Tray for the Convalescent | 113 |
| Rice Jelly with Fruit Sauce | 128 |
| Fruit Blanc Mange | 128 |
| First Step in making Orange Basket | 129 |
| Orange Basket | 129 |
| Orange Jelly in Sections of Orange Peel | 144 |
| Christmas Jelly | 144 |
| Wine Jelly, made to represent Glass of Lager Beer | 145 |
| Macedoine Pudding | 145 |
| Irish Moss Blanc Mange | 160 |
| Marshmallow Pudding | 160 |
| Charlotte Russe | 161 |
| Almond Tart | 161 |
| Small Ice-Cream Freezer and Substitutes | 176 |
| Cup St. Jacques | 177 |
| Flowering Ice-Cream | 192 |
| Ice-Cream in a Box | 193 |
| Frozen Egg Custard | 193 |
| Grape Fruit | 208 |

## LIST OF ILLUSTRATIONS.

| | FACING PAGE |
|---|---|
| Melon garnished for Serving | 208 |
| Orange Pulp | 209 |
| Orange prepared and arranged for Serving | 209 |
| Orange Mint Cup | 224 |
| Oat Wafers Mixture, illustrating Shaping | 225 |
| Oat Wafers | 225 |
| Wheat Crisps | 240 |
| Angel Drop Cakes | 240 |
| Sponge Basket | 241 |
| Stuffed Tomato Salad | 256 |
| Celery and Grape Fruit Salad, served in Green Pepper | 256 |
| Asparagus Salad | 257 |
| Tomato Basket, with Peas | 257 |
| Canary Salad | 264 |
| Harvard Salad | 264 |

# FOOD AND COOKERY

FOR THE

## SICK AND CONVALESCENT.

---

### CHAPTER I.

#### FOOD AND ITS RELATION TO THE BODY.

FOOD is that which builds and repairs the body, and furnishes heat and energy for its activities. Metabolism includes the processes by which food is assimilated and becomes part of the tissues, and the excretion of broken-down tissues as waste products. The body, by the analysis of its different organs and tissues, is found to contain from fifteen to twenty chemical elements, of which the principals are: carbon (C), $21\frac{1}{2}\%$; hydrogen, (H), $10\%$; oxygen (O), $62\frac{1}{2}\%$; and nitrogen (N), $3\%$. Phosphorus (P), sulphur (S), iron (Fe), chlorine (Cl), fluorine (Fl), calcium (Ca), potassium (K), sodium (Na), magnesium (Mg), and silicon (Si) are some of the others present. The elements found in the body must be supplied by the oxidation and utilization of the food stuffs, and the health of the individual will suffer if these are not properly maintained.

Food adjuncts are such substances as stimulate the appetite without fulfilling the requirements of food. Examples: tea, coffee, spices, flavoring extracts, condiments, etc., etc.

While air is not classified as a food, it is essential to life. Combustion cannot take place without it, and all food must be oxidized (which is a process of slow combustion) before it can be utilized by the body.

## CLASSIFICATION OF FOODS.

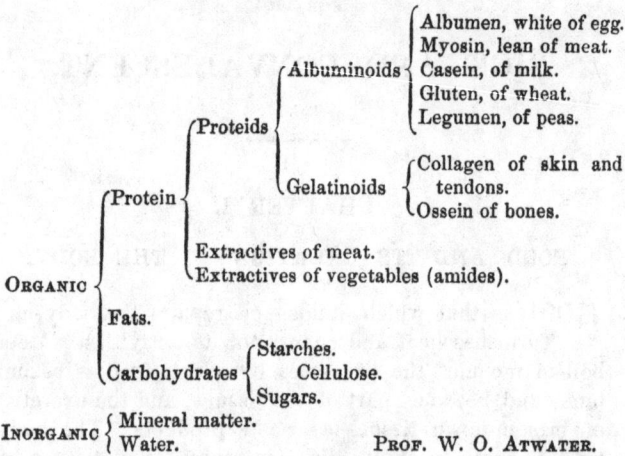

PROF. W. O. ATWATER.

The chief office of proteids is to build and repair tissues, and they only can do this work. They also furnish heat and energy, and in cases of emergency are capable of supplying fat. The chemical elements found in proteid foods are carbon, hydrogen, oxygen, nitrogen, sulphur, and generally phosphorus and iron. They differ from the other food principles inasmuch as they contain nitrogen, and nitrogen is essential to life.

The principal animal proteids are meat, fish, eggs, and cheese; the principal vegetable proteids are cereals, peas, beans, and lentils. The proteids obtained from animal foods are more easily digested and more completely absorbed than those obtained from vegetable foods. This is due in part to the presence of the large quantity of cellulose in vegetables. During the oxidation of proteids ammonia is set free, which neutralizes the acids constantly being formed.

The waste products of proteids are excreted by the urine in the form of urea. While a well-balanced dietary

## CLASSIFICATION OF FOODS.

contains all the food principles, it is possible to sustain life on proteids, mineral matter, and water.

Proteids are the most expensive foods, and there is often found to be an insufficient quantity in dietaries, especially among the poorer classes. It is conceded to be true, that in the United States with those of large incomes there is a tendency to an excess of proteids, but this does not apply to the average American family. Our people eat more than any other people, and do correspondingly more work. The growing child suffers more from the lack of proteid than the adult, as much material is required for building as well as repair. Until recently it was supposed that metabolism went on much faster in young cells, but now the greater activity of the child is held responsible for these rapid changes.

The chief office of carbohydrates is to furnish heat and energy and store fat. They contain carbon, hydrogen, and oxygen, the hydrogen and oxygen always being in the proportion to form water ($H_2O$).

Starch, the chief source of carbohydrates, abounds throughout the vegetable kingdom, being obtained from seeds, roots, tubers, stems, and pith of many plants. Examples: cereals, potatoes, sago, tapioca, etc.

Sugars, the other source from which carbohydrates are obtained, are classified as follows: —

Sucroses
(Disaccharids)
$C_{12}H_{22}O_{11}$
- Cane sugar (Sucrose).
- Beet sugar.
- Maple sugar.
- Malt sugar (Maltose).
- Milk sugar (Lactose).

Glucoses
(Monosaccharids)
$C_6H_{12}O_6$
- Grape sugar (Dextrose).
- Fruit sugar (Lævulose).
- Invert sugar (Honey best example).

HUTCHISON.

Carbohydrates include the cheapest kinds of foods and are apt to be taken in excess. In institutions where large numbers are fed there is a tendency in this direction.

Carbohydrates in the form of starch furnish a bulky food; and while a certain amount of bulk is necessary, an excess causes gastric disorders. Sugar is oxidized and absorbed more readily than starch. The monosaccharids are ready for absorption, dextrose being the sugar found in the blood. Some sugar is absorbed through the walls of the stomach, and this holds true of no other foods except alcohol and a very small per cent of peptones (proteids). No water is absorbed through the walls of the stomach.

Sugar (sucrose), on account of its cheapness and complete absorption when taken in combination and moderation, makes a desirable quick-fuel food. Milk sugar (lactose) is equal in nutritive value to cane sugar. Being less sweet to the taste and more slowly absorbed it is often used to advantage for infant feeding and sick-room cookery, where expense is not considered. The usual retail price of milk sugar is about thirty cents per pound. Milk sugar, under ordinary conditions, does not ferment and give rise to an excess of acids.

Sugars are more rapidly oxidized than starches. The former may be compared to the quick flash of heat from pine wood, the latter to the longer-continued heat from hard wood.

The starches furnish the necessary bulk to our foods and are also proteid sparers. Proteids give such an intense heat that but for the starches much of their energy would be wasted.

The waste products of carbohydrates are carbon dioxid ($CO_2$) and water ($H_2O$), which leave the body through the lungs, skin, and urine.

The fats and oils also furnish heat and energy, and constitute the adipose tissue of the body. Examples: Fats of meat, butter, cream, olive oil, etc. They are an expensive concentrated fuel food, yielding two and one-fourth times as much energy as an equal weight of carbohydrates. To those who do not consider expense in feeding, there is a strong tendency to increase the use of fats and oils and decrease the carbohydrates, while

## CLASSIFICATION OF FOODS.

in many respects they are interchangeable. "In the diet of children, at least, a deficiency of fat cannot be replaced by an excess of carbohydrate; and that fat seems to play some part in the formation of young tissues which cannot be undertaken by any other nutritive constituent of food," is a prevailing belief among competent observers.

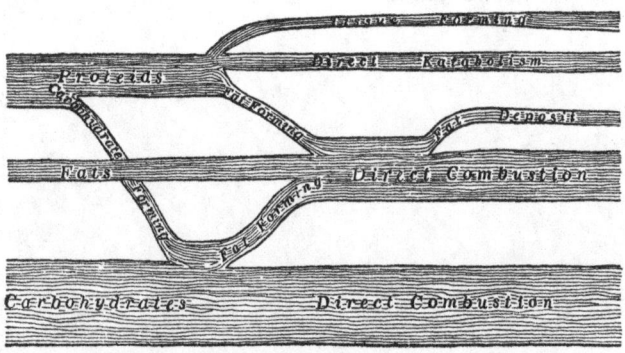

Showing how proteids, fats, and carbohydrates are split up in the body.

Water constitutes about two-thirds of the weight of the body, and enters into the composition of all the tissues and fluids. To keep the necessary proportion, a large quantity needs to be ingested. One of the great dietetic errors is the neglect to take a sufficient quantity. The amount found in foods is insufficient, and about five cupfuls should be taken daily in beverages. A vegetable diet diminishes the need of water, while one composed largely of animal food increases this need.

Mineral matter is necessary for the building of tissues, being found, principally, in the bones and teeth. It aids in the digestion of foods, and also assists in the diffusion of the fluids of the body. Phosphate of lime, or calcium phosphate, is the mineral basis of bones. Potassium, magnesium, sodium, and iron are minerals, all of which are essential to life. They usually enter the body in organic compounds. Sodium chloride (NaCl), common salt, is found in all tissues and secretions of the body except the enamel of the teeth. A sufficient quantity is obtained from our foods for the body's need; the average person, however, takes an additional quantity as a condiment, thus stimulating the appetite and increasing the flow of gastric juice.

## CHAPTER II.

### ESTIMATES OF FOOD VALUES.

THE familiar comparison between the body and the locomotive engine serves as a most forcible illustration for studying the fuel value of foods.

Food furnishes fuel to supply heat and energy for the body as wood and coal do for the locomotive. The food not only does this work, but it must also build and repair the human structure, while the locomotive is not capable of making its own repairs.

Latent heat is just as surely found in meat or bread as in wood or coal. They are both waiting to be oxidized, that they may be converted into heat and energy. As different kinds of wood and coal are capable of giving off different degrees of heat, and also giving off that heat in longer or shorter periods of time, so different food stuffs work in comparatively the same way.

The subject of the fuel value of food is of such great importance that within the last few years much time has been devoted to experiments along this line, and the results have furnished much valuable knowledge to aid us in correct feeding.

The latent energy in different foods has been determined by their oxidation, outside the body, in the apparatus known as the bomb calorimeter. Still further experiments have been made with the respiration calorimeter. By this apparatus not only is the fuel value of all the food taken into the body determined, but the excreta, products of respiration, and heat given off by the body are measured. From this statement it can be seen that man himself is used in making the experiments.

Results have shown that the oxidation of foods is the same in the body as outside the body.

"The amount of heat given off in the oxidation of a given quantity of any material is called its 'heat of combustion,' and is taken as a measure of its latent or potential energy." The calorie is the unit measure of heat used to denote the energy-giving power of food, and is equivalent to the amount of heat necessary to raise one kilogram of water 1° C. or about one pound of water 4° F.

1 gramme [1] proteid furnishes . . . . . . . 4 calories
1 " carbohydrates furnishes . . . . . 4 "
1 " fat furnishes . . . . . . . . . . 8.9 "
*Bulletin No.* 142 *U. S. Department of Agriculture.*
1 gramme alcohol furnishes . . . . . . . . . 7 calories

While proteids are capable of furnishing heat and energy as well as building and repairing tissues, it must always be remembered that their chief office is for the latter work. It is impossible for metabolism to go on without the production of some heat. The proteids are the only foods that contain nitrogen.

To determine the amount of nitrogen in a given food stuff, divide its grammes of proteid by 6.25. One gramme nitrogen equals 6.25 grammes proteid. The excretion of nitrogen for a man of average weight is about twenty grammes daily, the same amount being consumed. When the quantity of nitrogen is increased, there is a corresponding increase of its excretion, thus establishing nitrogenous equilibrium.

[1] 28.3 grammes equal 1 oz.

## Table showing Calorie Value of some Important Foods.

|  | Household Measure. | Avoirdupois. | Metric. | Calories. |
|---|---|---|---|---|
| Egg | 1 | 1½ oz. | 45 gms. | 75 |
| White of one egg | | 1 oz. | 30 gms. | 14 |
| Yolk of one egg | | ½ oz | 15 gms. | 56 |
| Milk | 1 cup | ½ pt. | 250 c c. | 170 |
| Cream, thin, 12% | 4 tablespoons | 2 oz. | 60 c.c. | 80 |
| Cream, thick, 18–20% | 4 tablespoons | 2 oz. | 60 c c. | 120 |
| Butter | 1 tablespoon | ½ oz | 15 gms. | 110 |
| Cheese | 1 tablespoon | ½ oz. | 15 gms. | 60 |
| Olive oil | 1 tablespoon | ½ oz. | 15 gms. | 135 |
| Sugar | 1 tablespoon | ½ oz. | 15 gms. | 60 |
| White bread[1] | 1 whole slice | 2 oz. | 60 gms. | 150 |
| Flour | 1 tablespoon | ¼ oz. | 8 gms. | 26 |
| Rice | 1 tablespoon | ½ oz. | 15 gms. | 50 |
| Rolled Oats | ⅓ cup | 1 oz. | 30 gms. | 116 |
| Boston crackers | 1 | ½ oz. | 15 gms. | 60 |
| Graham crackers | 1 | ⅓ oz. | 10 gms. | 40 |
| Beefsteak | 1 portion | 4 oz. | 120 gms. | 160 to 300 |
| Lamb chop | 1 | 1½ oz. | 45 gms. | 50 to 150 |
| Chicken | 1 portion | 3⅓ oz. | 100 gms. | 100 to 125 |
| Bacon | | ½ oz. | 15 gms. | 90 |
| Halibut | | 2 oz. | 60 gms. | 70 |
| Oysters | ½ cup | 5 oz. | 150 gms. | 75 |
| Beef juice | 2 tablespoons | 1 oz. | 30 gms. | 7 |
| Potato | medium size | 3⅓ oz. | 100 gms. | 100 |
| Banana | medium size | 3⅓ oz. | 100 gms. | 100 |
| Peach | medium size | 4 oz. | 120 gms. | 30 |
| Orange | medium size | 5 oz. | 150 gms | 50 |
| Orange juice | 2 tablespoons | 1 oz. | 30 gms. | 15 |
| Apple | medium size | 5 oz. | 150 gms. | 60 |
| Strawberries | 1 portion | 4 oz. | 120 gms. | 40 |
| Canned Tomatoes | 2 tablespoons | 1 oz. | 30 gms. | 7 |
| Prunes, dry | | 2 oz. | 60 gms | 175 |
| Breakfast Cocoa | 1 tablespoon | ¼ oz. | 8 gms | 36 |
| Brandy | 1 tablespoon | ½ oz | 15 gms. | 45 |
| Whiskey | 1 tablespoon | ½ oz. | 15 gms. | 45 |
| Sherry | 1 tablespoon | ½ oz. | 15 gms. | 15 |
| Liebig's Beef Extract | 1 teaspoon | | | Insignificant. |

[1] In ordinary computations entire wheat bread can be reckoned as having the same nutritive value as white bread.

1 lb. white bread furnishes 1215 calories: 1 lb. entire wheat bread.

FOOD AND COOKERY.

A man of average weight (one hundred and fifty-four pounds, or seventy kilos), at moderate work, requires about three thousand calories daily. The standard dietaries include one hundred and twenty-five grammes proteid, fifty grammes fat, and five hundred grammes carbohydrates.

| | | | | |
|---|---|---|---|---|
| Proteid | 125 grammes | $\times 4$ | = | 500 calories |
| Carbohydrates | 500 " | $\times 4$ | = | 2000 " |
| Fat | 50 " | $\times 89$ | = | 445 " |
| Total calorie value | | | | 2945 " |

### Table showing Number of Calories required under Different Conditions.

A man at light work . . . . . . . 2450 to 2800 calories
"   "   " medium work . . . . . . 2800 to 3150 "
"   "   " hard muscular work . . . 3150 to 4200 "
"   "   " rest . . . . . . . . . . 2100 to 2450 "

A woman needs eight-tenth as much food as a man.

The quantity of food required in a temperate and warm climate is about the same; the kinds, however, vary. Mother Nature, always wise and unerring, produces different crops to meet different needs. In our own country oats is grown in the northern part, rice in the southern.

In a cold climate more food is needed, — a fact not due to the temperature, but to the greater activity of the inhabitants, — and fat forms a larger proportion of the diet, as it is oxidized slowly in the body.

1140 calories. The same statement applies to many of the flours, thus: —

1 lb. flour furnishes 1665 calories.
1 lb. entire wheat flour furnishes 1675 calories.
1 lb. corn meal furnishes 1655 calories.
1 lb. corn starch furnishes 1675 calories.
1 lb. wheatlet furnishes 1685 calories
1 lb. hominy furnishes 1650 calories.
1 lb. granulated corn meal furnishes 1665 calories.
1 lb. wheat germ furnishes 1695 calories.
1 lb. tapioca furnishes 1650 calories.

A tall, thin person consumes more food than a short, stout person, for the reason that the larger surface exposed is the cause of a greater loss of heat.

Age has a marked effect upon the rations needed. A child from three to five years old requires four-tenths as much food as a man at moderate work; from six to nine years, one-half as much; while a boy of fifteen years requires as large a quantity as a man of sedentary habits.

The abuses of diet in youth are responsible for much suffering which develops later in life. The laws of retributive justice may be slow, but are, nevertheless, sure. Again, many of the diseases which occur after middle life are due to the habit of eating and drinking such foods as were indulged in during the early years of vigorous manhood.

In advancing years, when growth has ceased and activity has lessened, food is oxidized more slowly; therefore, a smaller quantity is required, and that in a form to be easily digested.

In arranging menus for individuals or families, personal idiosyncrasies must be considered. It is a homely saying, but true, that, "One man's meat is another man's poison."

The "Dietary Computer," by Mrs. Ellen H. Richards, is of great value to one whose desire it is to make out bills of fare according to food values. By its use money spent for foods could be used to better advantage, families would be better nourished, and disease would be less frequent.

## CHAPTER III.

### DIGESTION.

FOOD, before it can be utilized by the body, must undergo many mechanical and chemical changes to render it capable of digestion, absorption, and assimilation.

*Digestion* is the conversion of insoluble and indiffusible substances into soluble and diffusible substances capable of being absorbed. *Absorption* is the taking up of the digested food by the blood-vessels and lymphatics and conveying it to the blood, by which it is carried to every part of the body. *Assimilation* is the taking up by the different tissues from the blood such material as they need for growth and repair.

Digestion is carried on principally by ferments, and these act by contact. Food is taken into the mouth, masticated by the teeth, moistened by the saliva, and coated by the mucin in the saliva, which makes it easy to swallow. The *saliva* is an alkaline fluid secreted by three pairs of glands, — the parotid, submaxillary and sublingual. Ptyalin, which acts in an alkaline medium, is the ferment found in the saliva. It has the power of changing starch to maltose and dextrose, but has no effect on proteids or fats. The flow of saliva is continuous, but greatest during eating, about three pints being secreted every twenty-four hours.

Thorough mastication is very important, that the food may be finely divided before passing on into the alimentary canal. If not well masticated it is retained in the stomach for too long a time, thus favoring the development of bacteria, which give rise to acid fermentation.

# DIGESTION.

Food is forced by peristaltic action through the œsophagus into the cardiac portion of the stomach, where it comes in contact with the gastric juice. The gastric juice is a fluid which contains hydrochloric acid (HCl) and three ferments *(enzymes)*, pepsin, rennin and lipase. The flow of gastric juice is intermittent, but about the same quantity is secreted, daily, as of saliva.

*Pepsin* acts upon proteid foods, changing some to albumoses and peptones, while by far the largest part is simply swollen in gastric digestion. Pepsin is the principal ferment which acts upon gelatin. *Rennin* is a milk-curdling ferment, *lipase* is a fat-splitting ferment recently discovered.

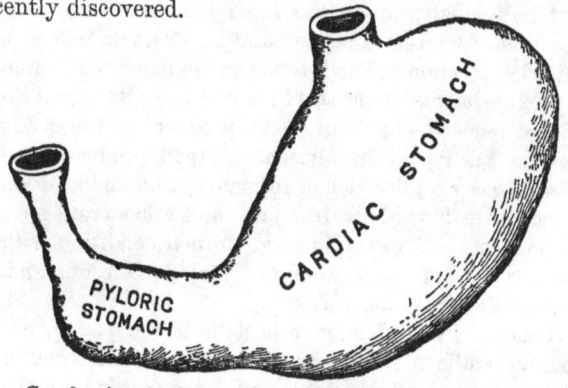

Cut showing the division of the stomach into two portions.

The digestion of starch continues for about one-half hour after entering the stomach; by that time the food material is sufficiently mixed with the gastric juice to render the whole acid, thus destroying the alkaline reaction. Fats are set free, and to some extent melted in the stomach. About six per cent of proteids, twenty per cent of sugar, and some salts are absorbed through the walls of the stomach. Water passes on with the partially digested food. If the food is liquid, the water leaves the stomach very quickly, and in drinking water some leaves the stomach before the last swallow is taken.

The stomach has two muscular motions. The first is a turning movement, which takes place in the larger or cardiac portion, mixing the food with the gastric juice, thus bringing the whole to a semi-fluid consistency.

The second is a wave-like movement which takes place in the pyloric end, by means of which the food is allowed to pass by intervals into the duodenum, which is the entrance to the small intestine.

The juice poured out in the pyloric portion contains no hydrochloric acid, but is neutral or slightly alkaline; pepsin is present.

The quantity of gastric juice varies not only in different individuals, but in the same individual according to the diet. Extremes in temperature exert an influence on gastric digestion. Pawlow has made many very interesting experiments along this line, and has discovered that a diet composed chiefly of meat produces a large flow of gastric juice poor in ferments; bread produces a small flow of gastric juice rich in ferments; while milk produces a moderate flow of gastric juice and a moderate amount of ferments. To keep in good normal condition without gain or loss of body weight, a plain, wholesome, mixed diet is the most satisfactory.

There is great danger, especially in the young, of becoming addicted to digestive habits. Each food calls forth a special gastric juice, and if the diet is limited to a few foods the power to assimilate others becomes lessened; therefore if the diet is increased, gastric disturbances are apt to occur. When a patient has been kept for some time on a milk diet, other foods must be introduced gradually, and in small quantities, for the comfort of the individual.

The stomach being capable of great distension, often gives rise to the taking of too much food at a single time. Three meals daily meet the needs of the average person. Dinner should be the heartiest meal, and should be served after the work of the day is over, when sufficient time may be allowed for eating, which may be followed by rest.

## DIGESTION.

In cases of impaired digestion, fifteen or twenty minutes is recommended for rest after each meal. Where a light breakfast is taken, a lunch should be indulged in in the middle of the forenoon. There are frequently found people of small stomach capacity who seem to require food at frequent intervals in small quantities; whereas if a meal is taken which would serve the needs of the average person, gastric disturbances follow.

Appetite has a marked effect on gastric digestion, and it is often necessary to stimulate the appetite. Attractive surroundings (plants, flowers, music, singing birds, etc.) are provided in institutions where money is not the first consideration. The sanitariums and hospitals in Germany are far in advance of ours in this respect. Good cooking plays a far more important part than surroundings, and it is the duty of the cook to stimulate the appetite by appealing to the sense of hearing, smell, sight, and taste.

While the stomach plays but a small part in digestion, the digestibility of foods is calculated by the length of time they remain in this organ. The average meal leaves the stomach in about four or five hours. The following table will be found of value in considering the ease or difficulty with which certain foods are digested.

### Table showing Time required for the Digestion of some Important Foods.

| KIND. | TIME. |
|---|---|
| Eggs, soft cooked (2) | 1¾ hours |
| Oysters, raw (3) | 1¾ " |
| Milk, one glass | 2 " |
| Graham Crackers (square) | 2 " |
| Rusks | 2 " |
| Beef, raw (3½ oz.) | 2 " |
| Eggs, raw (2) | 2¼ " |
| Cauliflower | 2¼ " |
| Bread, stale (2½ oz.) | 2⅓ " |
| Potatoes, baked (2) | 2 to 2½ " |
| Sweetbread | 2 to 3 " |

| Kind. | Time. |
|---|---|
| White Fish (Cod excepted) | 2½ to 2¾ hours |
| Tapioca, Arrowroot, and Sago Gruel | 2⅔ " |
| Beef, roast, rare | 3 " |
| Lamb Chops (3½ oz.) | 3 " |
| Chicken | 3 " |
| Game | 3 " |
| Apple, large (raw) | 3¼ " |
| Peas | 4 " |
| Beans | 4 " |

Digestion principally takes place in the small intestine. The stomach acts as a reservoir for food, playing but a small part in digestion. Many instances are recorded where people have been well nourished after the removal of the stomach. There was, however, a radical change in the diet, the food being taken in a liquid or semi-solid state.

Food in the small intestine comes in contact with two fluids, — the pancreatic juice and the bile (which is poured out from the liver), both of which are alkaline fluids. The flow of pancreatic juice is suspended except during digestion, while the flow of bile is constant but greatest during digestion.

The pancreatic juice contains four ferments, — amylopsin, trypsin, steapsin, and invertin.

Amylopsin acts upon starches and completes their digestion. Trypsin completes the digestion of proteids. Its action is similar to the action of pepsin in the gastric juice, but it is able to act in an alkaline medium. The proteids which were simply swollen in the stomach are now penetrated by this juice and their digestion is completed. Steapsin splits the fats into glycerine and fatty acids. The fatty acids combine with an alkaline solution and form soap. The bile salts also play an important part in the digestion of fats, but affect neither proteids nor carbohydrates. They, too, combine with fatty acids to form soap, and soap forms an emulsion. Fats thus emulsified are ready for absorption. Invertin acts upon cane sugar, changing it to levulose and dextrose.

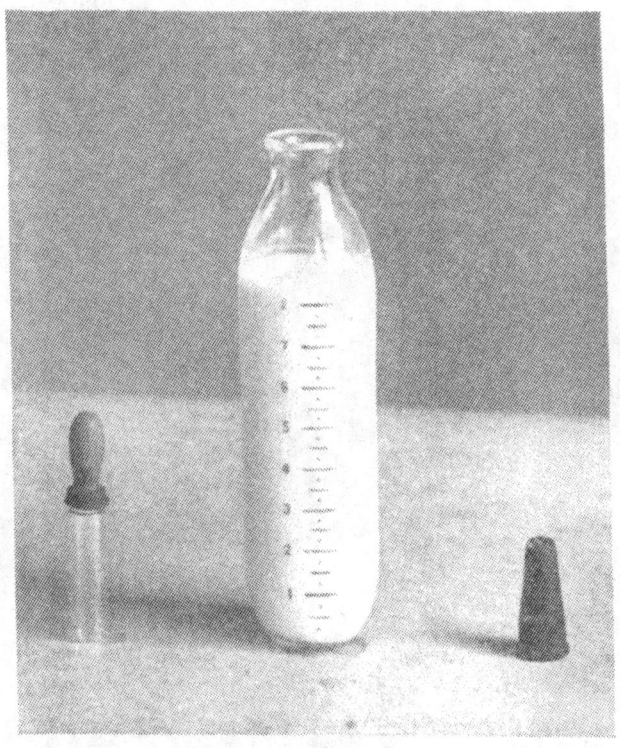

INFANT'S WATER BOTTLE, NURSING BOTTLE, AND NIPPLE

See p. 26

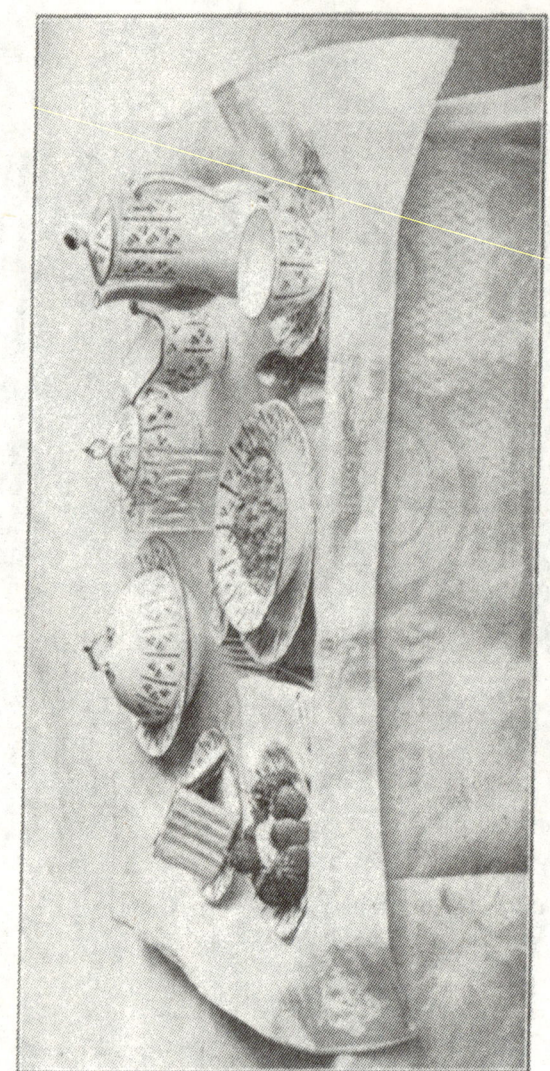

BREAKFAST TRAY
See p. 36

The liver acts as a storehouse for the body, to be called upon as needed. Some of the carbohydrates which during digestion have been converted into sugar, on reaching the liver are changed into glycogen, and glycogen is reconverted into sugar before entering the general circulation.

The digested food is now ready for absorption, although, as has been stated, the digestion of all foods need not be completed before the absorption of some foods take place. For example, alcohol, sugar, and some proteids and salts are absorbed in the stomach.

Food is moved along from the small to the large intestine by peristaltic muscular contraction. Absorption takes place to a small extent in the small intestine, but to a much larger extent in the large intestine.

Bile salts, on account of their great value, are nearly absorbed before reaching the rectum, and are used over and over again. Salts, bile pigments, connective tissue, and cellulose are not digested (although some authorities affirm that the cellulose in young vegetables is partially digested); these, with the waste products of metabolism, are excreted through the rectum as fæces.

## CHAPTER IV.

## FOOD AND HEALTH VERSUS DRUGS AND DISEASE.

DR. OLIVER WENDELL HOLMES is reported to have said, "I can count on the fingers of one hand the drugs commonly used by the general practitioner." Drugs are used at the present time to a less extent, and administered in smaller doses, than ever before. The physician of to-day knows that the recovery to health from disease is a natural process, and administers drugs to assist nature rather than to effect a cure. The study of foods and their effect on the individual is of equal importance to the study of drugs.

All infectious diseases are due to bacterial action. Germs enter the system in different ways.

1. Through the blood, — by inheritance.
2. Through the skin, — by bruising or bites.
3. Through air passages.
4. Through the lungs.

Drugs do not kill bacteria; exception must be made, however, to the valuable discovery of anti-toxins, which have done so much for the advancement of medical science.

The healthy person is constantly coming in contact with disease germs, but he is immune from the disease of which they are the cause, as anti-toxins are constantly being formed within the body which neutralize the poisonous effects of the germs.

Health may be defined as a sound mind in a sound body. The necessary conditions for health are: —

1. A correct supply of food.
2. The proper cooking of same.

3. Air and sunlight supply.
4. Good environment.
5. Exercise.
6. Rest.
7. Sleep.
8. Bathing.

It is safe to state that two-thirds of all disease is brought about by errors in diet, — either the food principles have not been properly maintained or the food has been improperly cooked. To one accustomed to visiting children's hospitals, or children's wards in general hospitals, this statement cannot seem an exaggeration, as the results of mal-nutrition are everywhere in evidence. Correct feeding should begin at birth, and continue through childhood, youth, manhood, and old age. Children more readily succumb to disease than older people; herein lies the necessity of paying the strictest attention to their nourishment and care.

"I have come to the conclusion that more than half the disease which embitters the middle and latter part of life is due to avoidable errors in diet, . . . and that more mischief in the form of actual disease, of impaired vigor, and of shortened life accrues to civilized man . . . in England and throughout central Europe from erroneous habits of eating than from the habitual use of alcoholic drink, considerable as I know that evil to be." — SIR HENRY THOMPSON.

The effect of foods on metabolism is a subject which has received much attention during the last fifty or sixty years. "Metabolism is the sum of the chemical changes within the body, or within any single cell of the body, by which the protoplasm is either renewed or changed to perform special functions, or else disorganized and prepared for excretion."

As early as the seventeenth century the idea was advanced that food furnished the necessary fuel for the body, but this theory attracted but little attention and seemed to be of almost no practical value as an aid to better living.

Towards the close of the eighteenth century oxygen was discovered by Priestley, which explained the process of combustion, which he believed to take place in the animal organism as well as outside the body. Liebig made valuable advances in the study of metabolism, and later investigations have verified the truth of his statements. In 1840 he published a dietary study which, from the standpoint of modern work, on account of its incompleteness, is of but little value. Still it was a pioneer publication which gave much assistance to many of his followers.

From 1850 to 1870 many experiments were made along these lines with animals, including cattle, dogs, and sheep. In 1865 and 1866 Voigt and Pettenkofer published the results of many experiments which they had made on man. To Voigt and his follows should be given the credit of the most valuable work of recent years.

Thorough work of a very high order has been done in Russia from which much accurate knowledge has been gained. The name of Van Noorden stands out prominently on account of his work on metabolism. Japan, Italy, Sweden, and England have all furnished students who have aided science along this line. As Americans we are especially proud of that which has been done in our own country. Chittenden and Flint have been earnest workers, and more accurate results are being obtained each year at the expense of our own government, under the able direction of Professor Atwater.

In the latest experiments account is taken of all food consumed, the excretory products, and the total energy manifested during the experiment, as heat or muscular work. The ideal has not as yet been reached, as no account has been made of body gain or loss, or the energy stored or transformed during the experiment.

## CHAPTER V.

### INFANT FEEDING.

IT would seem that every child's birthright should be a healthy mind in a healthy body, but man is not yet wise enough and science has not opened its doors sufficiently wide to render perfect living possible. Still searching for new truth, each year adds its part towards the complete solution, and "It is a proper or improper nutriment which makes or mars the perfection of the coming generation."

The power of the baby to grow mentally and physically must depend chiefly on its feeding, — although air and sunlight supply, environment, rest, sleep, exercise, bathing, and clothing all play a part not to be overlooked.

A young baby is a young animal, and must eat, sleep, and use some muscular effort in kicking and crying (at least one-half hour each day), to expand the chest and gain strength. A baby should be handled but little, and kept as quiet as possible. Much sleep is necessary, for during sleep the child develops and grows. For the first month a child requires sleep from twenty to twenty-two hours daily; three months, eighteen to twenty hours; six months, sixteen to eighteen hours; one year, fourteen to fifteen hours. A child gets the best sleep in a darkened, well-ventilated, quiet room; for during sleeping hours there is a subconscious activity, and if there is light and noise present the nervous, muscular, and tissue growth are hindered. Avoid the use of too much or too heavy clothing or covering, as either is a hindrance to the best growth and development.

The average weight of a child at birth is seven and one-seventh pounds for a male, while a female weighs about seven pounds. Many children have greater weight at birth, while still others weigh less; in either case the children are likely to be healthy. A child loses in weight for the first three or four days, but should regain its birth weight by the end of the second week; then there should be a constant increase of body weight, which should be in proportion to the original weight. The weekly gain should be from five to eight ounces until the fifth month, and from that time until the twelfth month the weekly gain is not as great, — about three and one-half to seven ounces. The child's birth weight should be doubled at five months and trebled at fifteen months. From these figures it can be seen that the most rapid gain is during the first five months. Regular increase in weight is the best and safest guide known for determining the health conditions of the child. Children do not gain as rapidly during the summer months, this being especially true during the teething period.

Nature has provided an animal food for the young of all mammalia, and mother's milk is the typical nourishment for her offspring in the early period of its existence. Statistics show that children among the slums of large cities will survive if fed from the breast, when if artificially fed, death is almost sure to follow.

The baby should be put to the breast six hours after birth; thus the secretion known as colostrum is injected, whose office is to cleanse the alimentary canal, thus preparing it for the milk secretion, which appears usually on the third day. After bathing and dressing, if the child lies quietly, it is left until the time of putting to the breast, but if it cries, one-half tablespoon of sterilized water is given at about 99° F., — the temperature of the child at birth. Children, like adults, need more water than is found in the food, and the baby should be given one-half tablespoon boiled water every four hours, after the second day, — the quantity being increased in proportion to the increase of the stomach capacity. It is best to have the baby drink it from a spoon, especially if it is to be fed

INFANT FEEDING. 23

from the breast; it is, however, generally easier for the child to take it from a small bottle with nipple attached. If the bottle is used, it is sometimes difficult to get the child to take the breast.

Regular feeding must be insisted upon as best for mother and child. It tends to keep the quality of the milk uniform, thus enabling the child to sleep better, not be overfed, and lessening the causes for indigestion. Too long intervals between the nursings produce a diluted product; while too short intervals, a condensed product. If regular feeding is observed the milk supply will agree with the capacity of the child's stomach. By more frequent nursing the milk glands are stimulated to secrete a larger quantity, and the little stomach capable of distension is overtaxed. Mothers should be made to realize that upon this care during a few months much of the later health and vigor of their offspring depend.

### Table for Infant Feeding.

| Age. | Number of Feedings. | Hours for Feeding. A.M. | P.M. |
|---|---|---|---|
| Birth to 2 months | 10 | 6 | 2 |
| | | 8 | 4 |
| | | 10 | 6 |
| | | 12 M. | 8 |
| | | | 10 |
| | | One Night-Feeding | |
| 2 to 3 months | 8 | 6 | 2 |
| | | 9 | 4 |
| | | 12 M. | 6 |
| | | | 8 |
| | | | 10 |
| 3 to 6 months | 6 | 6 | 3 |
| | | 9 | 6 |
| | | 12 M. | 10 |
| 6 to 12 months | 5 | 6 | 3 |
| | | 9 | 6 |
| | | 12 M | |
| 12 to 16 months | 4 | 7.30 | 2.30 |
| | | 11.30 | 5.30 |

# FOOD AND COOKERY.

That the baby may not be overfed, it is necessary to emphasize the stomach capacity at different ages; thus the following table may be of value: —

### Stomach Capacity.

At birth . . . . . . . . . . . . $\frac{5}{6}$ to 1 oz.
At 4 weeks . . . . . . . . . . . $2\frac{1}{2}$ oz.
At 8 weeks . . . . . . . . . . . $3\frac{1}{5}$ oz.
At 12 weeks . . . . . . . . . . $3\frac{1}{2}$ oz.
At 16 weeks . . . . . . . . . . $3\frac{56}{100}$ oz.
At 20 weeks . . . . . . . . . . $3\frac{3}{5}$ oz.

A mother's first thought should be for the welfare of her child, and she should wisely regulate her exercise and sleep, making an effort to control emotions and avoid nervous disturbances, which so readily affect the composition of the milk. A plain, wholesome diet, including meat, eggs, fish, cereals, fresh vegetables, and fruit, is recommended. Highly seasoned foods, pastry, and an excess of sweet foods should be avoided. Milk, or a beverage of which the principal constituent is milk, should be taken. While tea and coffee are not prohibited, cocoa is much more desirable. Oftentimes the three meals prove insufficient, and a luncheon may be introduced in the forenoon, and milk or gruel before retiring.

If the mother's milk proves inadequate to the child's needs, it often may be made suitable by change of diet and proper exercise. A child will lose on too rich a food as well as one lacking in nutritive value. The proteid and fat in human milk are subject to variations, while the mineral matter and milk sugar are nearly constant.

To increase the supply of milk, increase the liquid in the diet. To decrease the supply (which is seldom necessary), decrease the liquid. To increase the amount of proteid, eat more meat and decrease the exercise; to decrease the quantity, eat less meat, increase the quantity of liquid, and increase the exercise. To increase the fat, increase the meat, and also fats in a readily digested form, and walk two miles daily. To decrease the fat, eat correspondingly less meat and fat.

Too much proteid, which is the result of a large amount of meat, in the diet with little exercise, causes constipation and colic. If the fat is increased with the proteid, diarrhœa and vomiting follow.

### Human Milk.

Composition.  Reaction slightly alkaline.

| | |
|---|---|
| Water | 87 to 88% |
| Fat | 3 to 4% |
| Milk sugar (lactose) | 6 to 7% |
| Mineral matter | .1 to .2% |
| Proteid | 1 to 2% |
| Caseinogen | .59% |
| Lactalbumin | 1.23% |

KÖNIG.

NOTE. — While human milk has a slightly alkaline reaction, it is also amphoteric. It will change red litmus paper blue; blue litmus paper red.

### Cow's Milk.

Composition.  Reaction slightly acid.

| | |
|---|---|
| Water | 86 to 87% |
| Fat | 4% |
| Milk sugar | 4.5% |
| Mineral matter | .7% |
| Proteid | 4% |
| Caseinogen | 2.88% |
| Lactalbumin | .53% |

KÖNIG.

By comparing the tables showing the composition of human and cow's milk, it will be seen that cow's milk contains more proteid and mineral matter and less sugar of milk, the fat and water varying but little. The calf grows faster than the baby, therefore needs more building material. The baby, having a relatively larger surface exposed, loses more heat.

The proteid of milk is composed of lactalbumin and caseinogen. Lactalbumin is soluble in water, and as there is a larger percentage of this constituent in human than in cow's milk, the former during digestion forms into succulent curds; while the latter, containing more caseinogen, forms into dense cheesy curds.

Cow's milk, to form a typical infant food, needs to be modified. In many large cities throughout the United States, laboratories, with accompanying farms in outlaying districts, have been established to furnish proper infants' food. While human milk is self-modifying, thus meeting the needs of the child in the different stages of its growth and development, its composition varies but little during the period of lactation.

The modification of laboratory milk needs to be changed from time to time according to a physician's formula, limewater being added to neutralize the acid present in cow's milk. Human milk is sterile, while cow's milk, in the hands of the consumer, contains many varieties of bacteria; therefore it was formerly thought advisable to sterilize the modified product; but sterilization has been largely superseded by pasteurization, and this is not deemed necessary or advisable, where fresh milk can be procured from a reliable source, except in cases of bowel trouble or in extremely hot weather.

A child should not remain at the breast for more than fifteen or twenty minutes at each feeding. Never wake a healthy baby during the night for feeding. It is sometimes necessary during the day, as a young child is quite liable to turn night into day; but by persistent effort this may be overcome before it is an established habit.

If for any reason the mother is unable to nurse her child, she must make a decision between a wet nurse and artificial feeding. Cow's milk is best adapted for artificial infant feeding, although in its composition it is not as nearly like human milk as the asses' or the mare's. Cows can be kept more easily under strict control than most animals, and when carefully stabled, fed, watered, and cleaned, produce a food which can be modified to meet the baby's needs. Durham, Devon, Ayrshire, and Holstein breeds are most satisfactory. Always procure milk from the herd rather than from a single animal. If the supply be obtained from a single cow, it is not uniformly as good quality, for an indisposition, fright, or worry of the animal affects the milk, and this in its turn reacts upon the child.

Among intelligent and care-taking mothers, home modification is being successfully employed, always under the direction of a physician. It has advantages over laboratory modification, namely: —

1. Less handling.
2. Shorter time from milking to consumer.
3. Gravity cream digests more readily than centrifugal cream.
4. Less handling renders pasteurization seldom necessary.

It is beyond the scope of this work to give formulas for home modifications, as it is plainly the work of the physician. Simply for illustration a formula corresponding very nearly to human milk has been procured from one who is an authority on infant feeding.

#### For Home Modification.

Procure milk, delivered in quart glass jars, that has been reduced to a temperature of 45° F. as quickly as possible after milking, and allowed to stand for cream to rise for six or eight hours. Pour off eight ounces of top milk, or take out with a small dipper which comes for the purpose.

A glass tube is sometimes used for syphoning off the lower part of the milk, leaving the top milk in the jar. In order to do this a graduate glass is necessary, to determine the number of ounces drawn off. This later process being more complicated, is less practical for home modification.

### How to syphon Milk.

1. Place jar several inches above graduating glass into which milk is to be drawn.
2. Put thumb over end of syphon having the shorter arm.
3. Fill syphon with cold water.
4. Introduce long arm of syphon into jar of milk, having syphon touch bottom of jar.
5. Hold graduating glass directly under short arm of syphon, withdraw thumb, and water will flow from syphon, then milk.

### Formula for Modified Cow's Milk, closely corresponding to Human Milk.

| | |
|---|---|
| Top milk (10% fat) | 8 oz. |
| Boiled water | 11 oz. |
| Lime-water | 1 oz. |
| Sugar of milk | 2½ tablespoons. |

This amount is sufficient for ten feedings, allowing two ounces for a feeding. As soon as modified, it should be put in ten sterile nursing-bottles, each being plugged with absorbent cotton, and kept in a cold place until needed, then heated by plunging bottle in cold water and allowing the water to heat, gradually, until the milk is luke warm, about 98° F.

In the home modification of milk, the sugar of the milk (lactose) should be dissolved in boiling water before being added to the remaining ingredients.

Bottles and nipples for infant feeding should be of the simplest construction, that, easily, they may be kept perfectly clean. As soon as baby has finished nursing, the nipple should be removed from bottle, and nipple and bottle thoroughly washed, then the bottle filled with water and the nipple immersed in water. Both should be made sterile each morning, when the number of feedings for twenty-four hours is prepared. The nipples should be allowed to remain in boiling water five minutes, and then immersed in cold water, to stand until needed.

### How to pasteurize Milk.

Put milk in sterile, small-mouthed glass bottles, stop with cotton batting or absorbent cotton, place bottles in wire basket, immerse basket in kettle of cold water, and heat water gradually, to a temperature of from 158° to 167°. Keep at same temperature thirty minutes. Remove bottles, cool quickly, and put in a cold place.

By this process almost all of the disease germs are killed; also those germs which produce souring; but the spores, which are not killed, will develop after a few days.

### How to sterilize Milk.

Proceed as in the pasteurization of milk, raising the temperature of the water to the boiling point (212° F ), and keeping at this temperature thirty minutes. Sterilization is an efficient method of destroying all germs, but alters the taste of milk, coagulates the albumen, destroys the fine emulsion of fat, and renders the casein less easy of digestion.

Sterilizers are on the market which simplify the process of sterilization, and their use is recommended where expense need not be considered.

## CHAPTER VI.

### CHILD FEEDING.

A CHILD fed from the breast is weaned, usually, from the eighth to the twelfth month, the time depending upon the health of both mother and child, as well as the season of the year. Unless compulsory, this change would better not take place during the summer months. Changes in diet should always be gradual ones, which is not the exception with the baby. Healthy children may be taught to drink from a cup or mug before taken from the breast, which will dispense with the use of the bottle. On the other hand, oftentimes ill or delicate children will not take sufficient nourishment in this way, and the bottle becomes a necessity for the welfare of the child. Baby not only eats better, but sleeps better, and keeps happier.

Some children are allowed to use the bottle at nap and bed time until two years of age. While this seems to many an over-indulgence to the child, it is sometimes recommended by physicians as the best course to pursue.

A healthy child of from eight to twelve months may be given a crust of stale bread, educators, rusks, Zwieback, and strained, well-cooked cereal diluted with milk. The necessity for an occasional drink of water, which was emphasized in infant feeding, must not be overlooked in child feeding.

From twelve to sixteen months a child requires four meals daily.

| Meals. | Times for Serving. |
| --- | --- |
| Breakfast | 7.30 A. M. |
| Lunch | 11.30 A. M. |
| Dinner | 2.30 P. M. |
| Supper | 5.30 P. M. |

If a child wakes very early, it may be given a crust of bread, a cracker, or a small quantity of milk, but not enough to take away the appetite for breakfast.

For breakfast, serve a cereal sprinkled with sugar (sparingly) and top milk. Well-cooked, strained oatmeal, hominy, or any of the wheat preparations may be used, and it is desirable to offer variety. A glass of milk should accompany this meal.

For luncheon, give strained cereal and milk, allowing three parts milk to one part cereal. In order that the child may have sufficient nourishment, pour off the upper half of quart jars of milk (top milk). In this way the necessary fat is supplied.

For dinner, serve a soft-cooked egg, or beef, chicken, or mutton broth thickened with strained rice or barley; either with a piece of stale bread spread with butter, followed by steamed rice with cream and sugar, steamed or baked custard, junket custard, Irish moss blanc mange, strained stewed prunes, or juice of one-half orange. When eggs are introduced into the diet for the first few times, give but one-half egg. This quantity may be easily digested, while a whole egg might cause gastric disturbance.

For supper, serve strained cereal and milk, same as for lunch. A child from sixteen to twenty-four months takes four meals, with the same hours for serving as the younger child, with some greater variety.

For breakfast, in addition to cereal, give "soft-boiled," dropped, or coddled egg. Scrambled egg, if cooked with a small quantity of butter, may be occasionally served. It is well at this age to introduce one egg daily into the diet.

For luncheon, give bread and butter, cracker, or cereal jelly with sugar and top milk in addition to the luncheon before served.

For dinner, mashed baked potato, beef juice, boiled rice, or macaroni may be added.

For supper, whole wheat or Graham bread spread with butter, stewed prunes, baked apple or apple-sauce, in addition to the supper before served.

Children over two years of age may begin to take fish, meat, vegetables, and fruits. White fish, broiled, steamed, or boiled, may be given in place of egg. Broiled lamb chops, broiled beefsteak, or rare roast beef, broiled or roasted chicken, or boiled fowl, are all suitable food, if introduced occasionally in small quantities. Spinach, asparagus tips, young tender string beans, and peas forced through a strainer, are all allowable. Fresh ripe strawberries, served with sugar, but not cream, may be eaten in the early part of the day, but should never be allowed after dinner. Blueberries and huckleberries had better not be introduced until after the fifth year, as they often act as irritants and give rise to summer complaints.

Some children express a desire for bananas, which may be satisfied if the fruit is scraped to remove the astringent principle which lies close to the surface. Many physicians think they are more easily digested when baked.

Cocoa, as well as milk, may be given as a beverage. The menu at this age is so varied, and the digestive powers of the child so increased, that strained cereals will no longer be necessary. Indian meal mush may now be taken, as well as the oat and wheat preparations; also the cooked cereal products, put up ready for serving.

Always avoid the use, in the dietary of a young child, of salted meats, pork, or veal, coarse vegetables (beets, carrots, turnips, etc.), cheese, fried foods, pastry, rich desserts, condiments, tea, coffee, beer, or any alcoholic stimulant, and iced water.

The child's craving for sweets is a natural one and should be gratified. This is accomplished in part by sugar served with cereal and desserts. Vanilla chocolate is a most desirable food, as well as sweetmeat, and if eaten at the close of a meal is beneficial rather than harmful. Perhaps no food containing albumen, carbohydrate, and fat is as well absorbed as chocolate. All the sugar is taken up, and there is a loss of only two per cent of the albumen, starch, and fat.

The injurious effects of pure chocolate and candy are

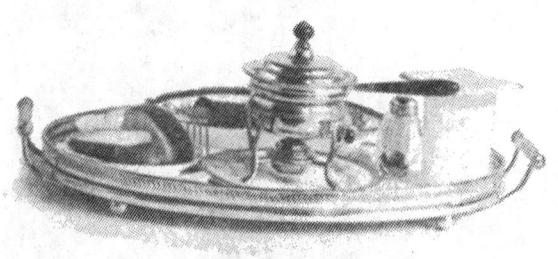

LUNCHEON TRAY
See p. 38

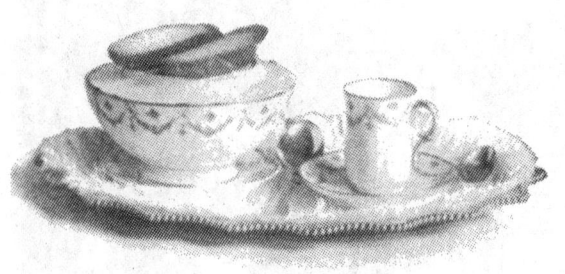

LUNCHEON TRAY
See p. 38

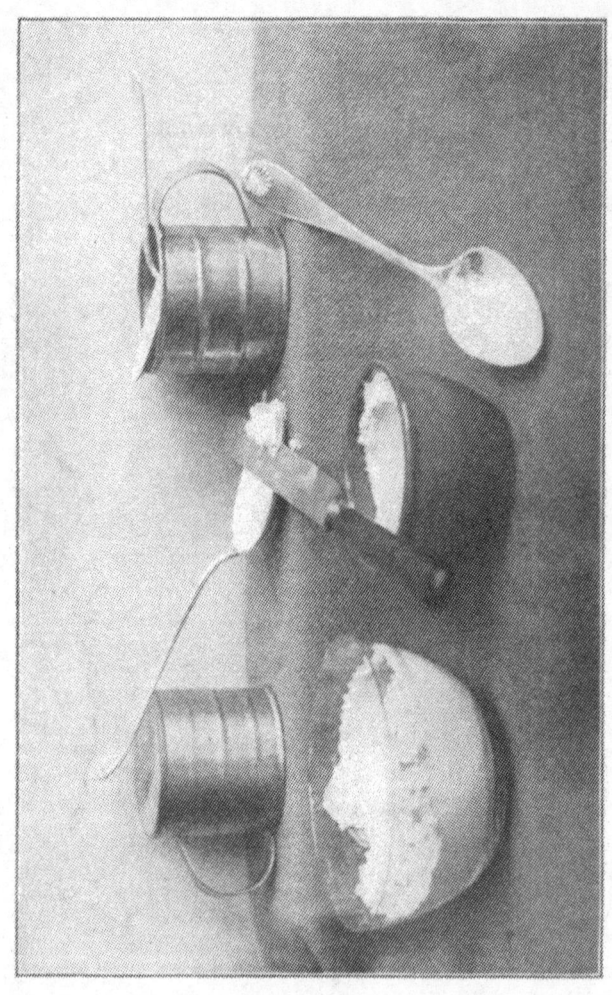

ONE-HALF PINT TIN MEASURING CUPS, AND TEASPOONS ILLUSTRATING THE MEASURING OF DRY INGREDIENTS due to their being eaten between meals or in excess, which destroys the appetite for plain, wholesome food.

When the time arrives that the nap is no longer needed, which time varies with different children, three meals usually suffice. The dietary may be gradually increased, until the child is able to partake of the family menu, avoiding, of course, a night dinner. The wise mother will encourage and continue a resting time until school hours interfere, even though not followed by sleep.

The food of the child at school is of equal importance to the food of the infant. It must not be forgotten that digestive processes go on quickly, and activity is so great in childhood that an abundant supply of well-cooked, nourishing food is essential for both the development of body and mind. The irritability and weak nervous condition of school children, which is often attributed to over-study, is more often the result of excitement, want of sleep, and malnutrition.

Never allow a child to go to school without a proper breakfast, of which a cereal served with sugar and rich milk or cream should form the principal dish.

Many children enter kindergarten at the age of three and one-half or four years, most of whom carry a luncheon, a few minutes being set aside for the purpose of eating the same. This luncheon should be very simple, and limited in quantity, that the appetite may not be destroyed for the hearty dinner. In many cases where a child is fortified with a good breakfast, the luncheon would better be omitted, as the child has a better appetite and enjoyment of the midday meal. In kindergartens attended by the poor, a luncheon is an absolute necessity to the child's welfare, and fortunate is the community where an appropriation is made for the supply of milk, with bread or crackers, or occasionally hot broth in the place of milk.

If the older child attends a one-session school, the luncheon must not be overlooked. Whatever else goes into the luncheon basket, sandwiches must hold first place. If a variety is introduced and pains are taken in their preparation, the little ones will look forward to them with as much interest as the sweets which follow. Doughnuts, rich cake, and pastry should be avoided, but simple crackers, cookies, and cakes may be used to advantage; also fresh and dried fruits and nuts. Figs, dates, and nuts have a high food value, and if well masticated, an active child will digest them with comparative ease.

In the high schools of many large towns and cities, lunch counters have been established for furnishing to the pupils well-cooked, nutritious food, at the least possible expense. Hot soups and cocoa may be found each day in addition to rolls, sandwiches, crackers, cookies, cake, fruit, and sometimes ice cream.

A child, relatively to his weight, requires more food than a man or a woman. Three considerations explain this necessity: —

1. The assimilative powers of a child are greater than those of an adult.
2. A child has a larger surface in proportion to his weight; which means a relatively larger heat loss.
3. A child is growing, therefore requires a relatively larger supply of building material.

### Table showing Amount of Food required for a Child as compared with a Man.

A child under 2 requires 0.3 the food of a man doing moderate work.

A child of 3 to 5 requires 0.4 the food of a man doing moderate work.

A child of 6 to 9 requires 0.5 the food of a man doing moderate work.

A child of 10 to 13 requires 0.6 the food of a man doing moderate work.

A girl of 14 to 16 requires 0.7 the food of a man doing moderate work.

A boy of 14 to 16 requires 0.8 the food of a man doing moderate work.

PROF. W. O. ATWATER.

## Table showing Increase of Calories required for a Growing Child.

| Age. | Proteid. | Fat. | Carbo-hydrates. | Calories. |
|---|---|---|---|---|
| years. | grammes. | grammes. | grammes. | |
| 1½ | 42.5 | 35.0 | 100 | 909.7 |
| 2 | 45.5 | 36.0 | 110 | 972.4 |
| 3 | 50.0 | 38.0 | 120 | 1050.4 |
| 4 | 53.0 | 41.5 | 135 | 1156.8 |
| 5 | 56.0 | 43.0 | 145 | 1224.0 |
| 8 to 9 | 60.0 | 44.0 | 150 | 1270.0 |
| 12 to 13 | 72.0 | 47.0 | 245 | 1736.8 |
| 14 to 15 | 79.0 | 48.0 | 270 | 1877.3 |

HUTCHISON, p. 453. SCHROEDER, *Archiv. für Hygiene*, iv. 39, 1886.

Children must have, for their best mental and physical development, a relatively larger proportion of proteid and fat in the dietary than their elders. The baby receives his proteid and fat from milk and cereals, but the older child needs, in addition to these, eggs, meat, and butter. Much of the pallor and stunted growth of some children is largely attributable to the lack of these very foods.

As carbohydrates furnish the cheapest form of food, they are almost never found wanting, and oftentimes are used to excess. Carbohydrate in the form of sugar, if injudiciously given, may prove harmful, but if used wisely, when it does not interfere with digestive processes, is a most useful fuel food.

The notion that sugar injures the teeth is largely a false one. If children are allowed to eat candy or cookies after the teeth have been brushed for the night, then the sweets which collect between them cause decay.

Milk, eggs, and meat are sources for furnishing mineral matter, but the chief value of fruit and vegetables lies in this food constitutent, upon which tissue growth so much depends.

## CHAPTER VII.

### FOOD FOR THE SICK.

THE feeding of persons in health is of great importance, but when one succumbs to disease, then feeding becomes a question of supreme moment. The appetite in health is usually a safe guide to follow, but is so perverted by disease conditions that it is unwise to consider its cravings. If these cravings are indulged, the food longed for is almost always a disappointment, as all things taste about the same, until the time of convalescence.

Never consult a patient as to his menu, nor enter into a conversation relating to his diet, within his hearing. The physician in attendance studies the symptoms so closely that he is able to determine what is required to meet the needs of the case. He orders nourishment given regularly, usually in small quantities, at frequent intervals. Appreciating the value of sleep, he never allows his patient to be awakened for feeding, unless the exigencies of the case create this demand.

In acute cases of disease, food plays a very important part towards recovery. The quantity and kind taken must vary greatly, according to the nature of the disease. Sometimes it proves expedient in cases of diarrhœa or dysentery to have the patient abstain for days from all food, except a very thin, starchy gruel, the object being to starve the germ which causes the disease; then, again, a patient, after a surgical operation, where there is a great loss of blood, needs a large supply of food.

Where the temperature is high, metabolism goes on so

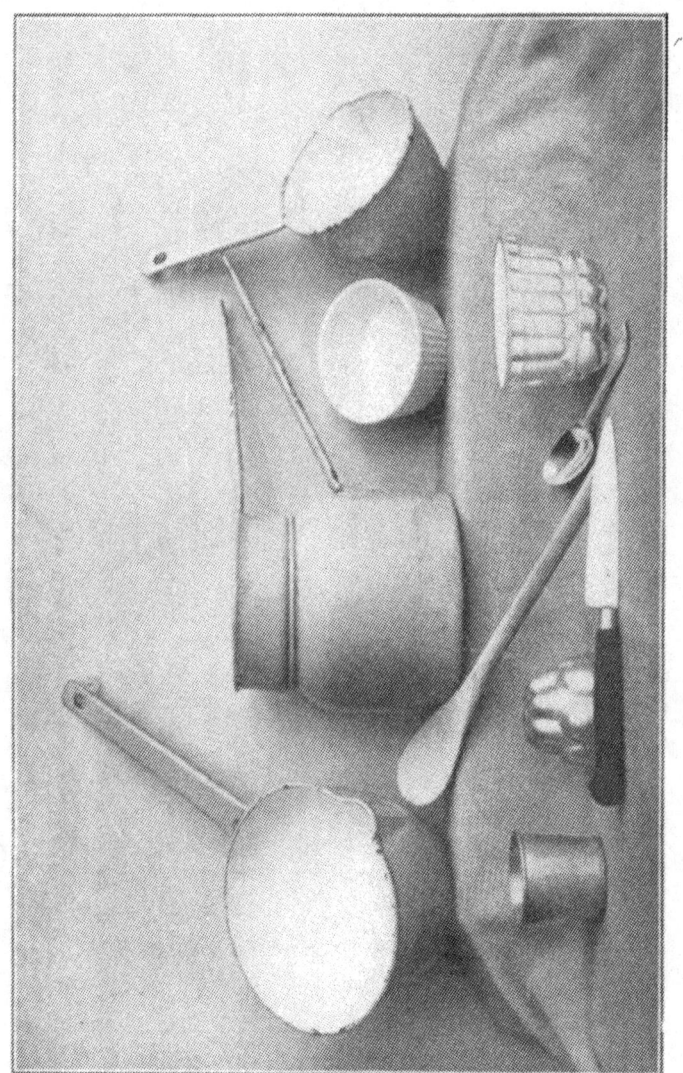

NECESSARY UTENSILS FOR INVALID COOKERY

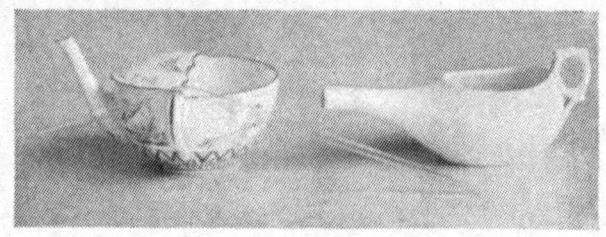

DRINKING CUPS AND GLASS DRINKING
TUBE OR SIPHON

See p. 62

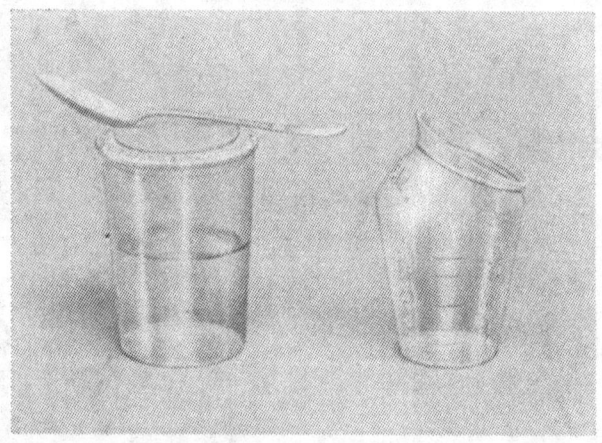

MEDICINE GLASS WITH GLASS COVER AND
IDEAL GLASS

See p. 62

easily digested food, usually in a liquid form. Water is given freely, to assist in carrying off the waste products.

In chronic cases, by a careful study of the food supply, much can be done to keep up the strength of the patient while endeavoring to overcome the disease. The greater the activity of the patient, the greater the need for food.

Personal idiosyncrasies in disease, as well as in health, play a very important part. Avoid giving food that will overtax the digestion or disagree with any of the conditions of the patient. Food must be assimilated to be of value. The teeth, the mouth, the stomach, and the intestines all must be considered. Some food, if well masticated, might easily pass from the stomach into the intestines, while if not masticated, might prove a stomach irritant. Some food that would not prove irritating to the stomach would cause fermentation in the intestines.

Many patients during the early stages of convalescence have an abnormally large appetite, which must be restricted, as over-feeding would prove dangerous; while with others the appetite needs to be stimulated.

Important things to consider in feeding the sick:

1. Appeal to the sense of sight.
2. Appeal to the sense of taste.
3. Consider temperature.
4. Digestibility.
5. Nutritive value.
6. Economy.

During the gradual return to a normal condition, through the long tedious hours of convalescence, the patient devotes much thought to when and what he shall be allowed to eat, and it is at this time that the taste is gratified as far as is advisable.

The best means of stimulating the appetite is to have good food, well cooked, and attractively served. The service should be the best at the command of the nurse, and too much attention cannot be given to every detail. The trays should be of correct size, so when laid not to have the appearance of being overcrowded; on the other hand, if a small amount is to be served, have a small tray. The tray cloth should be spotless, and just fit over edge of tray. If the correct size is not at hand, one should be folded to fit tray, or a napkin may often be utilized for this purpose. Select the choicest china, silver, and glassware, making changes as often as possible. It often proves pleasing to carry out a color scheme. Nervous patients are apt to be depressed in the early morning, therefore for this reason make the breakfast tray as attractive as possible by using bright flowers.

In setting a tray after laying the tray cloth, locate the plate. Place the knife at the right of plate, sharp edge toward plate. Place the spoon at the right of knife, bowl up. Place the fork at the left of plate, tines up. A bread and butter plate or individual butter is placed over fork a little to the left. The napkin is always placed at left of fork; then cup and saucer at right of spoon, with cup so placed that it may be easily raised by handle. The water glass is placed over knife at little to right. Arrange the other dishes to suit the convenience of the patient.

All eating is very much influenced by the taste. Some foods, easy of digestion, if repugnant to a patient, prove indigestible.

The temperature of food has a marked influence upon digestion. As a rule, hot foods should be served hot, cold foods served cold; but this often must be varied according to the case. Under certain conditions very cold or very hot food might retard digestion, thus increasing the amount of energy necessary for absorption.

Coarse foods, like Graham bread, some cereals, and vegetables containing much cellulose, pass through the alimentary canal so quickly that much of their nutritive value is lost, as so large a portion escapes absorption.

## FOOD FOR THE SICK.

Sugar is completely absorbed by the system, while starch holds second place. The proteid of meat and eggs is well absorbed, only three per cent being lost; in milk the loss is eight per cent. Fat, when taken in the form of butter, is almost completely absorbed, while in the absorption of fat in the form of milk, eggs, and cheese, there is a loss of six per cent; in the fat of meat, a loss of seventeen per cent. Bacon furnishes an exception to this rule, as it ranks next to the fat of butter and cream.

The nurse should be a student of the classification of foods, their fuel value and digestibility, thus being able to determine and regulate the needed rations for her patients.

In feeding the sick, strict economy should be considered only when necessary. That which the patient really needs should be furnished always, if possible. Even in homes where the income is limited, there is a general self-denial for the one who is ill. It is a too-frequent error to over-indulge a patient, for it weakens rather than strengthens. From this fact, together with lack of knowledge and appliance, those who are treated and cared for in a fine hospital are very apt to recover more quickly than those treated and cared for at home.

In hospitals, where large numbers are to be fed, many of whom are not able to contribute towards the support of the institution and still others who cannot pay their proportionate part, strict economy in food supplies becomes imperative. Many cheap foods are equally nutritious to the more expensive ones, and if well cooked and served are gratifying to all the senses to which one wishes to appeal.

In hospitals the dietaries are classified by the doctors, to assist the nurses in caring for their patients, as house, soft solid, soft diet, and liquid.

1. House, including: — soups, meat, fish, eggs, cereals, vegetables, fruit, desserts, etc.
2. Soft solid, including: — creamed sweetbreads, eggs, creamed toast, asparagus, baked custards, etc.

3. Soft diet, including: — soft-cooked eggs, milk toast, junket, boiled custards, jellies, etc.
4. Liquid, including: — broths, beef extract, beef tea, milk, gruels, egg-nogs, cream soups, cocoa, etc.

A special diet is such as is ordered by a physician for an individual case.

# CHAPTER VIII.

## COOKERY FOR THE SICK.

COOKERY is the art of preparing food for the nourishment of the human body. Cookery is the effect produced on food by the application of heat, air, and moisture.

"Uncivilized man takes his nourishment like animals, — as it is offered by nature; civilized man prepares his food before eating, and in ways which are in general the more perfect the higher his culture. The art of cooking, when not allied with a degenerate taste or with gluttony, is one of the criteria of a people's civilization." There are comparatively few foods that are at their best when taken in the raw state; they neither taste so good nor are they so easily digested as when subjected to some kind of cooking.

Disease is oftentimes due to improper feeding. The food rations have not contained the correct proportions of the food principles, or the food stuffs have been improperly cooked. " Food well cooked is partially digested."

### Objects of cooking Food.

1. To make more palatable.
2. To develop flavor.
3. To render more digestible.
4. To destroy bacteria and parasites.

### Methods employed for Cooking for the Sick.

1. Boiling . . . . . By heated water, 212° F.
    Simmering, 185° F.
2. Steaming . . . . . By vapor
3. Broiling  
4. Roasting  } . . . . By radiant heat and combustion of gases.
5. Baking

## FOOD AND COOKERY.

The subjects of food and feeding now stand on a scientific basis, and more attention is being paid each year to the subject of cookery. While the fact is to be recognized that there are some born cooks, the large majority need teaching and training. Cookery should form a part of every woman's education, and is especially important for those who have the feeding of the present generation, both in health and in disease.

For the best results in cookery, good materials, accurate measurements, care in combining ingredients, and a knowledge of the object to be attained are essentials. In cooking, the effect of heat at different temperatures and the time of exposure of different foods to such temperatures must be thoroughly understood to reach the best nutritive and economic results.

Measuring cups of glass, granite, or tin ware, divided into thirds or quarters, should be used. Tea and table spoons of regulation sizes, and also a case-knife, are indispensables. To insure uniformly good results, level measurements have been adopted by the leading teachers of cookery, which seem at the present time the best guide that can be given to the average cook. Perhaps the time may come when measurement by weight will be practical, and then accuracy will be assured beyond a doubt.

### Table of Measures and Weights.

A few grains . . . . = less than ⅛ teaspoon.
3 teaspoons . . . . . = 1 tablespoon.
14 tablespoons . . . . = 1 cup.
2 tablespoons sugar . . = 1 ounce.
2 tablespoons butter . . = 1 "
4 tablespoons flour . . = 1 "

To measure a cupful of any dry ingredient, fill cup, rounding slightly, using spoon or scoop, and level with a case-knife. Care must be taken not to shake the cup.

To measure a cupful of liquid, pour in all the cup will hold.

COOKERY FOR THE SICK. 43

To measure butter, pack solidly into cup and level with case-knife.

To measure a tea or table spoon of dry ingredients, dip spoon in same, fill, lift, and level with a case-knife, the sharp edge of knife being towards tip of spoon. Divide with knife lengthwise of spoon for half spoonful; divide halves crosswise for quarters, and quarters crosswise for eighths. Less than an eighth of a teaspoon is considered a few grains.

To measure tea or table spoons of liquid, dip spoon in liquid and take up all the spoon will hold.

To measure tea or table spoons of butter, pack butter solidly into spoon and level with a knife. Divide same as for dry ingredients.

Measure and have at hand all ingredients necessary for the preparation of a dish before attempting to combine.

### Ways of combining Ingredients.

1. STIRRING.
    Employed to mix ingredients.
    A circular motion, widening the circles until all is blended.
2. BEATING.
    Employed to enclose air.
    A turning of ingredient or ingredients over and over, continually bringing the under part to the surface, thus allowing the utensil used to be brought constantly in contact with the bottom of the dish and throughout the mixture.
3. CUTTING AND FOLDING.
    Employed to so mix ingredients that air already introduced may not escape.
    A repeated vertical downward motion with a spoon and a turning over and over of mixture, allowing bowl of spoon each time to come in contact with bottom of dish. These motions are alternated until thorough blending is accomplished.

The application of heat for boiling or steaming is not difficult to understand. Broiling and roasting need more care, while baking requires good judgment, coupled with experience. In the many cook books, various oven tests are suggested, and oven thermometers have been placed upon the market, but all are of but little practical value, as one must gain this knowledge by her own experience.

Vegetable foods abound in starch. Cold water separates starch grains; boiling water causes them to swell and burst.

*Experiment 1.* Mix two tablespoons flour with one-third cup cold water, and let stand five minutes. Flour settles to bottom of vessel.

*Experiment 2.* Stir mixture and heat to boiling point. Starch grains swell and burst, making a paste.

Dry heat, at a temperature of 320° F., changes starch to dextrine, which is soluble in cold water. Examples: Crust of bread and baked potato.

In cooking vegetables the object is to soften cellulose as well as swell and burst starch grains, and this is best accomplished by keeping the water at the boiling point throughout the entire cooking. By the proper cooking of starchy foods their digestibility is greatly increased.

Albumen is the principal constituent of white of egg. It is dissolved in cold water, and coagulated by heat at a temperature of 134° to 160° F.

*Experiment 1.* Put white of egg in cold water, stir, and albumen is dissolved.

*Experiment 2.* Put white of egg in cold water, heat gradually to boiling point, and albumen coagulates.

One of the proteids of meat is albumen, some of which is soluble in cold water and coagulated by heat.

*Experiment 1.* Cut beef in small pieces, put in cold water, and let stand twenty minutes. Water of a reddish color.

*Experiment 2.* Heat to boiling point and dissolved albumen will be coagulated.

*Experiment 3.* Cut beef in small pieces and plunge into boiling water. Albumen will be coagulated quickly, thus preventing its escape.

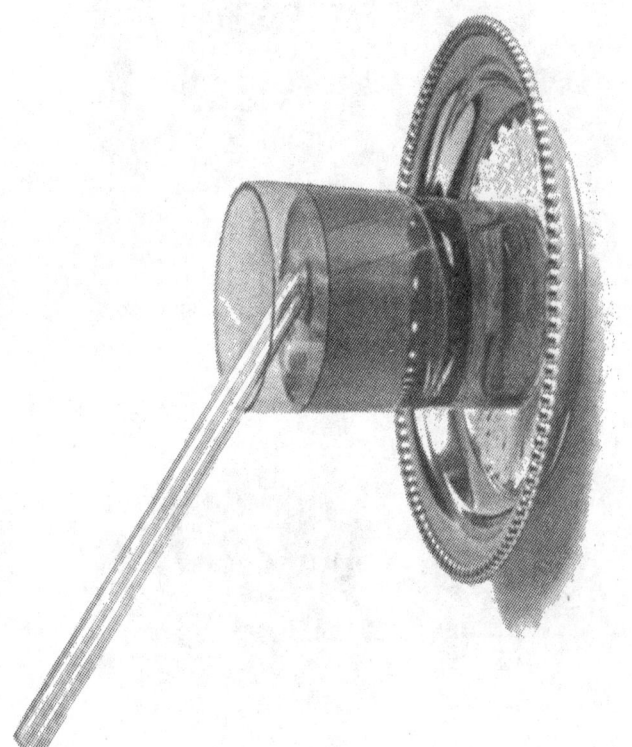

CURRANT JELLY WATER
See p. 69

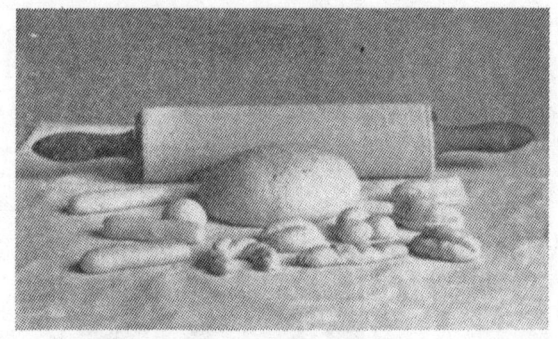

BREAD DOUGH WITH SUGGESTIONS FOR SHAPING
See p. 62

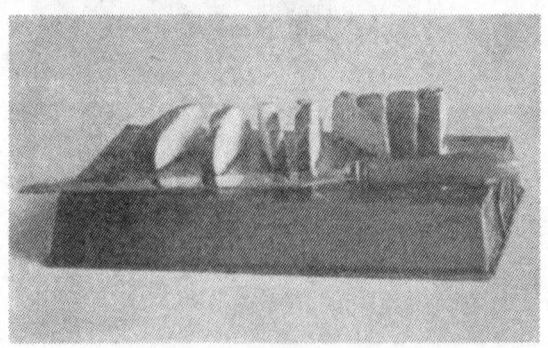

ZWIEBACK
See p. 97

In using meats for soup-making, the object is to draw out as much of the goodness as possible. This is accomplished by putting the meat on in cold water, and allowing the water to heat gradually to the boiling point, then simmering for several hours, after which time the meat is deprived of its extractives, some mineral water, and soluble albumen, though the greater part of its nutritive value is not extracted; nevertheless, lacking flavor, it is hardly palatable for serving. In the making of stews, when meat and broth are both to be used, the meat should be put on in cold water, brought quickly to the boiling point, and then allowed to simmer until tender.

Experiments have shown that where the water is allowed to boil vigorously during the entire cooking, the connective tissue has been gelatinized, while the fibres are hard and indigestible; quite the reverse is true of the fibres where the meat is cooked for a longer time at a lower temperature, and the connective tissues are partially dissolved. In the latter case the economy of fuel is worthy of consideration.

Cold water dissolves albumen, hot water coagulates it, as does intense heat. Meats, when broiled or roasted, are brought in direct contact with intense heat (coal, gas, or electricity furnishing the fuel), and turned frequently, thus searing the entire surface as quickly as possible. This method is applied to the more expensive cuts of meat. Meat, when baked in a hot oven, is commonly called roasted, as the old method of roasting before live coals has almost passed out of use.

In cooking meats, when the object is to retain as much nutriment as possible, the surface should be subjected to a high temperature to quickly coagulate albuminous juices. When cooked in water, the water must be at the boiling point to accomplish this, allowed to boil vigorously for five minutes, and then allowed to simmer for several hours. This method is applied to the cheaper cuts of meat.

## CHAPTER IX.

### WATER.

MORE than two-thirds of the weight of the body consists of water. An adult requires five pints daily, and is furnished with this supply from the food he eats and the beverages he drinks. The outgo is even greater than the income, owing to the chemical changes which are constantly taking place in the body.

Pure water is composed of hydrogen and oxygen, there being two parts of hydrogen to one part of oxygen. The symbol of water is $H_2O$.

Water as found in nature is never chemically pure. It not only contains many mineral substances, but decaying animal and vegetable matter, and often pathogenic germs. From this statement it may be seen that a water supply cannot be too carefully guarded.

The clear, colorless, tasteless fluid furnishes the average person with sufficient evidence of its purity; while if lacking in any of these qualities he seems to be equally assured of its unfitness for consumption. These tests are entirely useless, and scientific investigations are the only safeguards to a proper water supply.

Filters, as used to render drinking water pure, are a delusion and a snare. The bed of a filter furnishes a desirable soil for the growth of bacteria, and while some of the larger organic particles are removed by filtration, the rapidity with which the micro-organisms increase render it less fit for use.

Distilled water, prepared for medicinal purposes, is chemically pure. It is flat and insipid to the taste, having been deprived of its atmospheric gases. When used as a beverage it should be aërated. Boiled water is freed from all organic impurities and salts of lime are precipitated.

Water for household consumption is derived from five sources: —
1. Rains.
2. Rivers.
3. Surface water and shallow wells.
4. Deep Artesian wells.
5. Springs.

In many large towns and cities a system of reservoirs has been built, fed by springs and streams which have greatly improved water supplies.

Where well water is used, especial attention should be given to the location of the well. It must be of sufficient distance from drains, cesspools, and barnyards to prevent contamination.

Water drawn from large ponds, lakes, or rivers having a bottom of rock, clay, or gravel, usually furnishes a safe supply. The law, nevertheless, requires frequent analyses — thus helping, as far as possible, to make healthful conditions prevail.

Water is frequently spoken of as hard or soft. Hard water contains mineral matter to a greater extent than soft water, the amount varying from eight to seventy grains to the gallon.

The hardness is due principally to salts of lime and magnesia. Soft water is free from an excess of these salts, containing but three to four grains to the gallon. Water is the greatest known solvent, and the softer the water the greater its solvent power.

### Water Temperatures.

| | |
|---|---|
| 32° F. | Freezing point. |
| 32 to 65° F. | Cold. |
| 65 to 92° F. | Tepid. |
| 92 to 100° F. | Warm. |
| 100° F. and over | Hot. |
| 185° F. | Simmering point. |
| 212° F. | Boiling point (sea level). |

## FOOD AND COOKERY.

Many people are accustomed to boil water for drinking purposes. Hard water, due to the presence of carbonates of lime, is rendered soft by boiling with a small quantity of bicarbonate of soda ($NaHCO_3$).

### Uses in the Body.

1. To quench thrist.
2. To nourish.
3. To regulate body temperature.
4. To assist in carrying off waste products.
5. To maintain the proper degree of dilution for all the fluids of the body.
6. To stimulate the nervous system and various organs.
7. To form a part of all cell life, as metabolism cannot go on without it.

Cold water to a small extent retards gastric digestion, but increases peristalsis. If a glassful is taken before breakfast and upon retiring, it often cures constipation.

Tepid water is successfully used as an emetic, 90° F. being the temperature at which it is administered.

Hot water acts as a stimulant to gastric digestion. It leaves the stomach more quickly and is more quickly absorbed than cold water. Hot water relieves thirst better than cold water. It will also relieve nausea, — a small quantity of crushed ice having the same effect.

Water has many uses of valuable importance to man which ought to be mentioned; namely, for transportation, manufacturing purposes, and the generation of electrical power; but the purpose of this work is to consider it as a cleanser, an antiseptic, and a source of infection. The relation which bathing bears to health need hardly be emphasized, as it has for so long a time been duly recognized. Frequent bathing keeps the pores of the skin open, thus enabling much waste matter to be eliminated. Water is a carrier of disease germs, and too frequent are the cases of typhoid fever caused by drinking water. The only sure way of destroying pathogenic germs

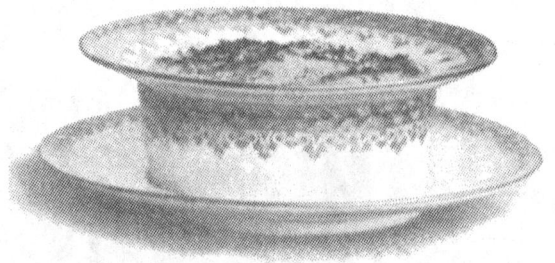

SHIRRED EGGS
See p. 111

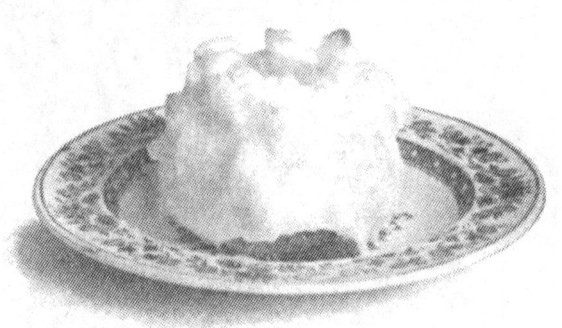

EGG IN A NEST
See p. 112

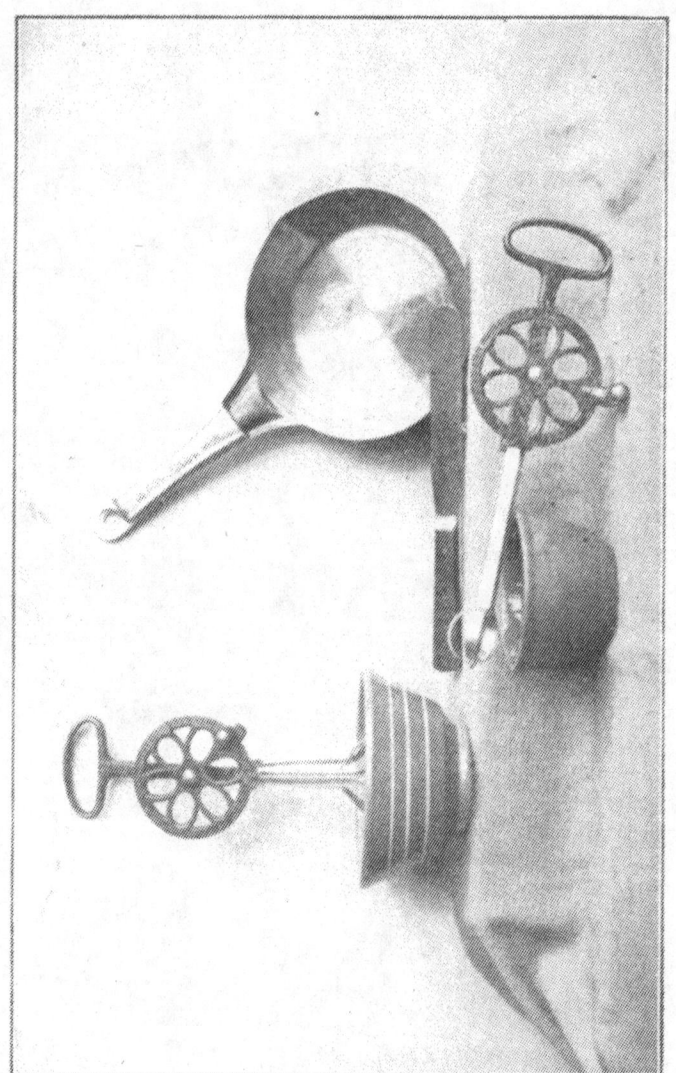

UTENSILS USED IN THE MAKING OF OMELETS

# WATER. 49

in water is by boiling the same. Boiled water is a valuable antiseptic, and will not ferment.

There are many charged, carbonated, and mineral spring waters bottled and put upon the market. Some are used as table beverages, others for medicinal purposes.

Ordinary water, artificially charged with carbon dioxid ($CO_2$), is called soda water, and may be purchased by the glass, usually in combination with fruit syrups or in syphons. Such water, when sold at the druggist's, contains a larger per cent of $CO_2$ than carbonated (naturally charged) waters, which renders it cooler to the taste, as the gas in passing off withdraws heat.

Plain soda water, taken in moderation, assists gastric digestion. It is a bad practice to indulge too freely in soda water with fruit syrups, as it causes a tendency to flatulency and indigestion. Almost all so-called fruit syrups are chemically prepared in the laboratory.

Among the most common carbonated table waters may be mentioned, Poland (uneffervescing), and Vichy, Johannis, Apollinaris, and Seltzer (effervescing). These often tempt people to drink who would otherwise neglect to do so, and in cases of fever they may be freely given. They are useful to dilute alcoholic liquors, and they are quite apt to relieve nausea and vomiting.

The alkaline mineral waters are all carbonated. Their most important ingredient is alkaline carbonates, and sodium chloride, sometimes sodium sulphates being present. Examples: Saratoga, Vichy, White Sulphur Spring, Hot Sulphur Spring, Hunyadi, and Londonderry Lithia Waters. Lithia water is often recommended in cases of rheumatism or gout; Hunyadi for liver troubles and indiscretions in diet.

Where patients are advised by physicians to visit water cures the good results obtained are due as much to change, rest, treatment, and quantity of water ingested, as to any especial value that the water itself contains.

## CHAPTER X.

### MILK.

MILK is an ideal food. This statement is plainly demonstrated by the fact that it furnishes the nourishment for the young of all mammalia during the period of their most rapid growth. While its value must not be overestimated in the dietary of the healthy adult, it is a matter of fact that in many countries the inhabitants live for the most part on it. This is true of the peasants of Norway, Sweden, and Switzerland, the Bedouins of Arabia, and the peoples dwelling in the mountain regions of Asia and on the pasture lands of the Sahara. It would be necessary for the man at work in the United States to consume four quarts daily in order to get the necessary quantity of proteid, and by so doing he would be furnished with an excess of fat and a limited supply of carbohydrates. No one food can meet all the requirements of the body except during infancy.

Milk should be regarded as a food rather than as a beverage. While it is a liquid outside the body, as soon as it enters the stomach it is made solid by the action of rennin, which causes it to become clotted. Milk is of most value in a mixed dietary, when taken between meals with a cracker or piece of bread, and it should be sipped rather than drunk. If taken quickly in large quantities, so dense a curd is formed in the stomach that it is with difficulty that the gastric juice acts upon it. As has been stated, each food calls forth a special kind of gastric juice, and in the case of milk it is in moderate supply and of moderate strength. Children absorb ninety-six per cent of the total solids of milk, while adults absorb eighty-nine per cent. With the aged, as digestion becomes impaired, milk should hold a prominent place in the daily dietary.

# MILK.

### Composition of Cow's Milk.

| | |
|---|---|
| Water, 86.90 | Proteids, 3.60 |
| Sugar, 4.80 | Fat, 4.00 |
| Mineral Matter, .70 | |

Many milk analyses have shown that the nutritive constituents of milk vary to a considerable degree, this even holding true of the milk from a single cow at different milkings, the greatest difference being in the quantity of fat. Jersey and Guernsey breeds yield the largest quantity of fat, but a smaller supply of milk. The largest amount of fat is obtained in the morning's milking.

The quality and quantity of milk is not only determined by the breed, but by the age, health, housing, feeding, care, and time of lactation of the animal from which it comes. It is an absolute necessity that the milk supply be carefully inspected, and in all large cities chemists are employed for this purpose, whose work has been of the greatest value.

Milk is more quickly contaminated than any other food product.

### How contaminated.

1. By improper feeding of animal.
2. " poor conditions due to nursing, worrying, etc.
3. " disease germs from the cow.
4. " extraneous disease germs.
5. " souring and decomposition.
6. " absorption of bad odors.

Milk, as soon as it comes from the animal, should be put in sterile vessels, cooled as quickly as possible, covered, and kept at a low temperature.

In the hands of the consumer it always contains a large number of micro-organisms, the greater number of which tend to increase lactic fermentation, which causes souring. If milk is kept under favorable conditions and for not too long a time, these do not sufficiently multiply to cause anxiety.

The pathogenic germs in milk are often causes of typhoid fever, diphtheria, scarlet fever, tuberculosis, and cholera. They are killed at 167° F., a much lower temperature than the micro-organisms which produce souring, and they also occur in smaller numbers.

When in doubt of the milk supply, it is always best to scald it.

If milk is allowed to stand for a few hours, the fat rises to the surface in the form of cream; this is due to its lower specific gravity. Such cream is called gravity cream. When a separator is used for removing cream, the cream thus obtained is called centrifugal cream. It must not be inferred from this that cream contains nothing but fat, for it holds relatively as large a proportion of sugar and proteid as milk itself, the deficiency being in the proportion of water. Cream is an expensive form of fat, and must be regarded as a luxury.

Lactose (sugar of milk) is equal in nutritive value to cane sugar. It has some advantages over cane sugar, for under ordinary conditions it does not ferment, it is not so quickly absorbed, and it is a diuretic. Lactose is not so sweet to the taste as cane sugar, which renders it of value in the sick-room; it is, however, an expensive fuel food.

The proteid of milk is the cheapest form in which animal proteid may be obtained. It consists principally of casein, albumen to a smaller extent, some globulin, and traces of peptone.

Potassium, sodium, calcium, magnesium, iron, sulphur, phosphorus, and chlorine are all found in the ash of milk in the form of oxides, chlorides, or acids.

### Skim Milk.

Milk from which most of the fat has been removed is known as skim milk. The quantity of fat removed depends on the manner in which the work is accomplished. Separator skimmed milk has less fat than that from deep cold setting. Skim milk has more proteid than whole milk, and a slightly larger proportion of milk sugar.

Skim milk may be advantageously used by the poorer classes. Its deficiency in fat may be made up, easily, by obtaining it from cheaper sources than whole milk.

### Buttermilk.

Buttermilk is obtained from cream during its manufacture into butter. Its composition differs but little from that of skim milk. It contains less proteid and sugar and more fat.

It has a slightly acid taste, which makes it an agreeable beverage, and it is well borne by people of weak digestion.

It acts as a laxative.

### Whey.

When milk is clotted by the action of rennet, wine, or an acid, and after standing a few minutes is strained through a double thickness of cheese cloth, the liquid obtained is known as whey. It is a slightly laxative fluid of small nutritive value.

### Koumiss, Kefir, and Matzoon.

Koumiss, originally fermented mare's milk, was first made, hundreds of years ago, in the steppes of Russia and Southwestern Asia. A double fermentation takes place in its manufacture, — lactic and alcoholic. Lactic fermentation begins first, while alcoholic lasts longer. It is the purpose of the Koumiss maker to hinder lactic fermentation as far as possible. Koumiss is made in the United States from cow's milk, yeast being the ferment used.

The alcohol ($C_2H_5OH$) and carbon dioxid ($CO_2$) formed during fermentation render the milk more easily digested and absorbed than in its natural state. It is consequently of great value in the sick-room, and is the one form in which milk seldom fails to be retained by the patient.

Kefir and Matzoon are fermented cow's milk, varying but little in composition from Koumiss. Koumiss and

Matzoon may be purchased in all cities and large towns of the leading druggists. Home-made Koumiss (p. 74) is most satisfactory.

### Ways of preserving Milk.

1. By scalding.
2. By pasteurization.
3. By sterilization.
4. By condensation.
5. By evaporation.

### Adulteration.

The adulteration of milk is far less frequent than formerly, as inspection, under law, is liable to take place at any time.

Where adulteration takes place it is accomplished, most commonly, by the removal of some of the cream or the addition of water. Salt, sugar, chalk, and starch are less often employed as adulterants. Annatto, caramel, or aniline dyes are used for coloring, that the product may look as though it were of the best quality.

Milk sours so quickly during warm weather that preservatives have often been resorted to to overcome this bacterial action. Among these have been found borax, boracic acid, salicylic acid, benzoic acid, potassium chromate, and carbonate of soda.

While these adulterants and preservatives are not poisonous when taken in the milk for an indefinite period, they are deleterious to health.

Massachusetts authorities prohibit the sale of "not of standard quality" milk as well as of adulterated milk; while other states have equally stringent laws. The following statute defines standard milk: —

"If the milk is shown upon analysis to contain less than thirteen per cent of milk solids, or to contain less than nine and three-tenths per cent of milk solids exclusive of fat, it shall be deemed for the purposes of this act to be not of good standard quality except during the months of April, May, June, July, and August, when milk containing less than twelve per cent of milk solids, or less than nine per cent of milk solids exclusive of fat, or less than three per cent of fat, shall be deemed to be not of good standard quality."

### Effects of Cooking.

When milk is heated a scum rises to the top, which consists of coagulated albumen, a small quantity of coagulated casein, and some fat. If the scum is removed some of the nutritive value of the milk is lost. If scalded milk is beaten with an egg-beater the scum, which is so unsightly, is well intermingled with the mass.

Milk should always be heated in a double boiler, where it never reaches a higher temperature than 196° F. If heated in a single utensil, it may reach the boiling point (214° F.), when it is liable to boil over or to burn, and it always takes an unnecessarily long time to wash and scour the dish.

The taste of milk is altered by the application of heat. The flavor of cooked milk is not so agreeable to the taste as uncooked milk. For this reason, if cooked milk is to be taken alone, it should be chilled as quickly as possible, which somewhat overcomes the change of taste.

### Digestibility.

Milk is easy of digestion and absorption. When comparing the digestibility of raw with cooked milk experiments have shown such different results that one cares to be guarded in making statements. The clots formed by cooked milk are smaller and less dense than those formed by raw milk; notwithstanding this fact, it is a prevalent belief that the casein is not so readily absorbed nor the fat so completely assimilated.

### Milk in the Sick-Room.

The value of milk as a food in cases of disease cannot be overestimated.

### Advantages.

1. It contains the five food principles.
2. It is inexpensive.
3. It is easily procured, measured, and taken.
4. It agrees with most people.
5. It does not overtax the digestive system.
6. It is a non-irritant.
7. It may be modified.
8. It may be combined with other foods.
9. It is deficient in uric acid derivatives.

### Objections to a strictly Milk Diet.

1. Its bulk.
2. Danger of insufficient nourishment.
3. Taste disliked.
4. It causes nausea (probably due to fat).
5. Forms dense clots.
6. Causes constipation (overcome by magnesia).
7. Increases acidity of urine.
8. Introduces micro-organisms.
9. Causes fur-coated tongue.

To the casual observer the disadvantages might seem to more than counterbalance the advantages. This is not the case, however, as the disadvantages in most cases may be easily overcome.

When whole milk does not agree with a patient, skim milk, or cream diluted with water, may often be employed successfully.

### Adapting for the Sick.

1. Altering taste.
    By heating, adding salt, pepper, ginger, cinnamon, nutmeg, tea, coffee, chocolate, lime-water, seltzer water, Apollinaris, beef extract, brandy, whiskey, rum, or sherry.

2. Improving digestibility.

By skimming, scalding, diluting with charged waters or farinaceous gruels, or by adding alkalines or acids. Addition of salt prevents biliousness.

Bicarbonate of soda prevents mal-fermentation. By the addition of farinaceous gruels milk forms in less dense clots.

By scalding, lactic acid fermentation is restricted. Hot milk soothes mucous membrane, allays a slight throat irritation, increases peristalsis, and tends to produce sleep.

3. Predigesting.

By adding Fairchild's Pancreatin or Pepsin powder, which changes the proteids to albumoses, and if the process is continued long enough, to peptones. If converted to peptones there will be a bitter taste.

Predigested milk is used in extreme cases to bridge the patient over a critical period, and for forced feeding in many hospitals and by many physicians.

According to the best authorities, however, predigested milk has no advantage over ordinary milk. From the fact that the proteids are partially digested, it would seem that a large amount of nutriment could be given in predigested milk; if, however, it is administered in sufficient quantities to supply a large amount of nutriment, one of two symptoms usually appear, — diarrhœa or nausea.

## CHAPTER XI.

### ALCOHOL.

ALCOHOL, $C_2H_5OH$ (ethyl alcohol), is obtained by the fermentation of sugar. It must be considered as a food, as it is so completely oxidized in the body, only ten per cent passing out of the system. The question of its use is a moral one, and in health it is entirely unnecessary. It does not enable a man to do more mental or physical work, and the higher sensibilities are not assisted. Armies and athletes always avoid its consumption.

*High proof* alcohol, as sold, contains ninety-five per cent of alcohol; while *absolute* alcohol contains ninety-nine per cent.

Alcoholic beverages are divided into

Fermented
- Ale, 3 to 6% Alcohol.
- Cider, 4% "
- Beer, 4 to 10% "
- Porter, 6% "
- Stout, 6% "
- Champagne, 9 to 12% "
- Red and white wines, 10 to 14% Alcohol.
- Exception, Sherry wine (17%).

Distilled
- Gin, 17% Alcohol.
- Brandy (Cognac), 40 to 47% "
- Rum, 40 to 65% "
- Whiskey, 44 to 50% "

When an extra quantity of alcohol is added, liquors are said to be fortified.

Distilled liquors are responsible for nine-tenths of the evil results of intemperance. The new and raw ones are the most harmful, for they contain a considerable quantity of fusel-oil, — a poisonous natural product difficult to eliminate. This diminishes with age, when they mellow and improve in flavor.

Alcohol is used in the sick-room for bathing purposes, and is usually diluted with water. Its local effect is that of an irritant.

Alcoholic beverages produce: —

1. Cheer and good fellowship.
2. Excitement and buoyancy.
3. Loss of self-control and judgment.
4. Loss of control of muscular movements.
5. Stupor.
6. Depression.

The physiological effects of alcohol are as yet incompletely understood. Its effect on the respiratory system is very slight, and on the circulatory system very doubtful; but it is given for the purpose of stimulating heart action. If given in small quantities it assists gastric digestion; in moderate quantities, it retards the flow of gastric juice; and in large quantities albumen is precipitated. Its effect on metabolism is that of partially paralyzing the cells, thus causing them to lose some of their power to break down proteids, carbohydrates, and fats.

Effects produced by the habitual use of alcoholic beverages: —

1. Throat becomes husky.
1. Chronic gastric catarrh.
3. Inability to resist disease.
4. Fatty degeneration of the liver and hardening of its cell walls.
5. Thickening of the walls of the arteries, especially the artery that supplies the heart. The heart, being improperly nourished, gives out, and heart failure is the result.
6. Apoplexy.

It should be left to the physician to dictate the kind, quantity, and frequency of administering alcoholic beverages. One kind is often given to advantage, while several might disturb digestion. They are preferably given before or at the time of meals. When taken between meals they should be accompanied by a biscuit or cracker.

### Conditions which justify their Use.

1. When the pulse is persistently weak.
2. When there is persistent high temperature.
3. When there is nervous exhaustion.
4. When there is tremor or low delirium.
5. When the digestive system fails to do its work.
6. When the aged are feeble or exhausted.
7. Cases of shock or accident.

The use of alcoholic beverages in some diseases seems almost imperative. Lives, without doubt, have been saved by the use of champagne. In fevers it is often given to produce depression, which results in sleep. In this way much strength is saved for the critical crisis. Brandy and red wines are given in cases of diarrhœa on account of the tannic acid they contain, which acts as an astringent. Erysipelas seems to be one of the diseases which calls for large quantities of alcohol. From eighteen to twenty ounces of brandy or whiskey may be administered daily without producing any intoxicating effects. Diabetes also demands the use of alcoholic stimulants. Brandy is the liquor generally preferred, as it assists in the digestion of fats. Pneumonia in feeble or elderly subjects calls for alcoholic stimulants; while in cases of diphtheria patients are often saved by their early and energetic use.

Many malt extracts and malted foods have been placed upon the market, some of which contain a minimum quantity of alcohol; but they are principally valuable for the diastase they contain, which aids in the digestion of carbohydrates.

## ALCOHOL. 61

The value of the patent spring medicines usually lies in the alcohol which they contain. Their stimulating effects lead many to believe that they are receiving permanent help rather than a temporary support. By analysis many have been found to contain as much alcohol as is present in sherry wine; while in others the per cent is greatly in advance. Would it not be wise to consult a physician rather than experiment along lines where danger is so imminent?

## CHAPTER XII.

### BEVERAGES.

A BEVERAGE is any drink. Water, the chief one of them all, is Nature's beverage. Almost all of the beverages have but little nutritive value (exception must be made, however, to egg-nogs, cocoa, chocolate, etc.); nevertheless their use in health as well as in disease should be carefully considered. When abstinence from solid or semi-solid food is necessary for a short time, a liquid diet must furnish the nourishment.

Starchy beverages include toast, rice, and barley water. Rice and barley water are given to reduce a laxative condition of the bowels, and are often used alternately. Rice water is soothing to the whole alimentary canal. Toast water is given in extreme cases of nausea.

Fruit beverages are cooling, refreshing, slightly stimulating, and are valuable for the salts, acids, and sugar they contain. They are frequently employed when high temperature is present. Lemons and oranges are most used in the making of fruit beverages on account of their cheapness and popularity. Raspberries, strawberries, pineapples, currants, grapes, and tamarinds are used less frequently. As all fruits contain one or more acids, a physician should be consulted as to the kind to be given in individual cases. Pineapple contains a ferment which digests proteids.

Wine whey is slightly stimulating, and is often retained in severe gastric troubles. For a limited period it may be used successfully for debilitated infants with weak digestion. It stimulates the digestive ferments to such an extent that there may be a gradual return to a regular diet. Clam water and oyster liquor sometimes stimulate the appetite. Clam water, administered in small quantities, is especially valuable in relieving extreme cases of nausea; in larger quantities it acts as a laxative.

Egg-nogs, and other beverages in which eggs are used, play a most important part in the dietary of the sick, for by their use nutriment in a concentrated form is easily administered.

### Tea.

The leaves of the evergreen shrub, Thea, furnish the tea of commerce, both black and green.

The best brands of black tea are imported from India and Ceylon; the best green tea comes from Japan, and a small quantity from China. Tea leaves before curing have neither odor nor flavor.

There are four gatherings annually. The first picking comes in April, and is considered the best.

Climate, elevation, soil, cultivation, selection of the leaves, and the care in the picking and curing of them, all go to make up the difference in quality. First quality tea is made from the young, tender, whole leaves. In black tea the leaves are allowed to ferment, while in green tea the leaves are unfermented.

Tea is a stimulant rather than a nutrient. Its stimulating effect is due to the alkaloid thein and a volatile oil. Its astringency is due to tannin. Black tea contains less tannin than green tea, while the thein and oil vary but little.

Tea should always be made as an infusion, by the use of freshly boiled water, with but one infusion to each measure of tea. The practice of allowing tea to boil, or allowing leaves to be used and reused with a small additional supply, cannot be too strongly condemned. The thein is so soluble that it is almost immediately dissolved out of the leaf. Tannic acid is developed as soon as tea is placed in boiling water, but in a small quantity. Experiments have shown that more tannic acid is developed in a five-minute than in a three-minute infusion, and the longer it stands, the more tannic acid is drawn out.

Tea drinkers require less food than those not addicted to its use, as it has been proved that there is less wear to the tissues when it is frequently indulged in. This accounts for the large quantity drunk by the poor. It would appear from its immediate stimulating and satisfying effects that it had a food value; but when it is constantly used to take the place of food, sooner or later evil effects are apparent, and the victim, if attacked by disease, finds that the system offers little resistance. The harmful effects are due, principally, to the tannic acid and oil, as thein stimulates rather than retards gastric digestion.

Tea is stimulating, refreshing, and often relieves bodily fatigue and headache. It has a slight influence in regulating circulation and temperature. It is one of the most cooling drinks in summer and warming drinks in winter. On an empty stomach it acts as a diuretic. Excessive tea drinkers are apt to become nervous, to suffer from insomnia and mental depression. The habit must be closely guarded, for the habitual, excessive tea drinker often becomes a nervous wreck.

To the aged it is "The cup that cheers." It certainly proves a useful stimulant as the functional activities of the stomach become weakened. It never should be given to children, and would better be avoided by the young.

### Coffee.

Coffee is the seed of the berry of the evergreen tree Caffœa Arabica, which yields, annually, three harvests. Each berry contains two seeds enclosed in a husk. Exception must be made to the male berry, which contains but one seed.

Coffee was formerly cured by being dried in the sun, but owing to the warm climate and frequent rainfalls in the countries in which it is grown, slow artificial heat is preferable, and is imported to be cleaned, sized, roasted,

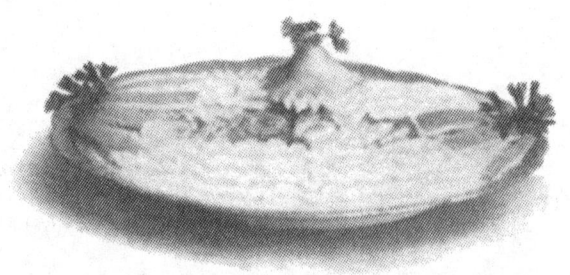

BROILED FISH, GARNISH OF POTATO BORDER
AND LEMON

See p. 129

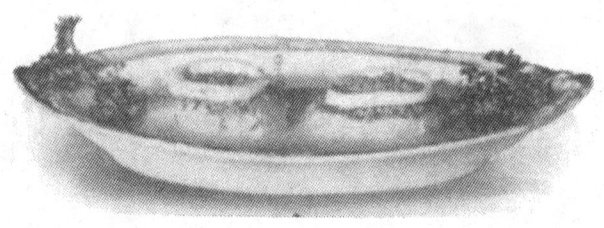

BAKED FILLETS OF HALIBUT

See p. 130.

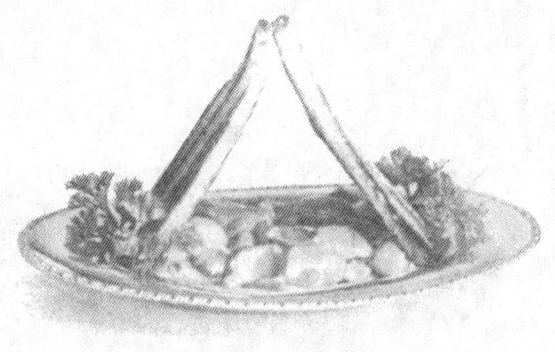

FANCY ROAST, GARNISHED WITH TOAST POINTS
AND PARSLEY
See p. 132

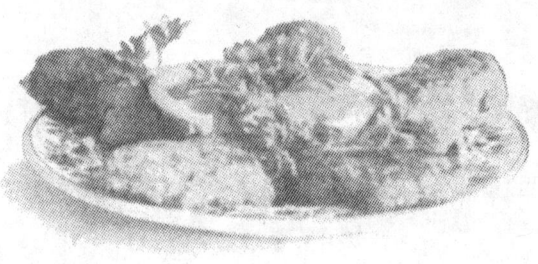

BROILED OYSTERS
See p. 133

and ground. The coffee berry in its raw state has no odor or flavor, both being developed by roasting.

For its cultivation it requires a warm climate, rich soil, and protection from wind and storms.

Java coffee is the finest coffee grown, but much sold under that name does not come, necessarily, from the island of Java. Any coffee having the distinctive flavor of Java coffee, no matter where grown, bears the name. Maleberry Java commands a higher price than any other coffee on the market. Brazil, Central America, Mexico, and Arabia are all coffee countries.

Coffee, like tea, is usually blended, the most popular mixture being three or four parts Java to one part Mocha. The Mocha gives a certain sparkle and acidity which the general public demands.

Coffee, like tea, is a stimulant. Its stimulating effect is due to caffein and a volatile oil. The effect of caffein is nearly identical with that of thein. Coffee also contains tannin. As taken for a beverage it is more stimulating than tea, from the fact that so much more is used. Its food value lies in the sugar and cream served with it.

Coffee should be bought in small quantities and kept tightly covered in a glass jar or tin canister. It should not be ground until purchased, and when convenient, it is best ground at home. On account of the large quantity of volatile oil it contains, it quickly depreciates in value.

Coffee may be prepared as a decoction (boiled coffee), filtration, or infusion. Coffee for filtering should be finely ground.

Coffee strengthens heart action, increases respiration, and excites mucous membrane. It is a nerve stimulant and a diuretic. It removes the sensation of fatigue, for which reason it is used by many nurses when on night duty. It is often valuable to relieve nausea after an anæsthetic, and often proves useful in cases of opium and alcoholic poisoning.

A cup of black coffee assists digestion, while a cup of breakfast coffee, as ordinarily served, retards digestion, but not to as great an extent as tea. When there is a flatulent state of the stomach, tea increases the amount of gas, in which case coffee is to be preferred. When taken in excess coffee produces biliousness, languor, restlessness, heartburn, palpitation of the heart, tremor, dyspepsia, and insomnia.

Many preparations have been put upon the market as coffee substitutes, but to the coffee drinker there is no substitute. They, however, make a pleasing hot beverage, and when properly made and served with sugar and cream, they have a food value. To the adult a single cup of coffee at breakfast and a single cup of tea at luncheon seldom prove harmful, and are acceptable to the average person.

### Cocoa and Chocolate.

Cocoa and chocolate are manufactured from the cacao bean of commerce. This bean, a native of Mexico, is the seed of a fruit from six to ten inches in length, containing from twenty to thirty seeds. The area of the cocoa belt for remunerative crops is limited, being chiefly confined to Mexico, South America, and the West Indies. The fruit matures throughout the year, taking four months for ripening; but the principal harvest is in the spring.

The fruit is gathered and allowed to remain in a heap on the ground for twenty-four hours, the pods are then cut open and the seeds removed, drained, and put in a sweating-box for two days to undergo the process of fermentation. The flavor of the bean depends largely upon the care taken during this process. Now the beans are dried in the sun, after which they are ready for exportation.

Having been exported in this crude state, they must be cleaned, assorted, and roasted; then the thin, brittle coverings removed by machinery. The thin coverings are sold under the name of *cocoa shells*. The broken roasted beans constitute *cocoa nibs*. *Chocolate* is the cocoa nibs crushed, pulverized, and moulded Vanilla and sweet chocolates have the addition of sugar and flavoring. In the manufacture of *cocoas* nearly one-half of the fat is removed from cocoa nibs.

Unlike tea and coffee, cocoa and chocolate, though slightly stimulating, have a food value which should not be overlooked.

### COMPOSITION.

|  | Proteid. | Fat. | Carbohydrates. | Mineral Matter. | Water. | Calorie Value per lb. |
|---|---|---|---|---|---|---|
| Chocolate | 12.5% | 47.1% | 26.8% | 3.3% | 10.3% | 2720 |
| Breakfast Cocoa | 21.6% | 28.9% | 37.7% | 7.2% | 4.6% | 2320 |

The stimulating effect of cocoa is due to theobromine, a principle closely allied to thein and caffein; it also contains some tannin.

Cocoa as a beverage may be used by many with whom tea and coffee disagree. There are some, however, who find it clogging and heavy on account of the large quantity of fat it contains. This is usually attributable to the fact that it is taken with a hearty meal. In cases of enfeebled digestion, cocoa usually agrees with the patient better than tea or coffee.

### Rice Water.

2 tablespoons rice.   3 cups cold water.
Few grains salt.   Cream or milk.

Wash rice by placing in strainer and allowing cold water to run through. Soak thirty minutes in cold water, heat gradually to boiling point, and let boil until rice is soft. Strain, reheat rice water, season with salt, and if too thick dilute with boiling water. Add milk or cream as the case may require.

### Barley Water.

2 tablespoons barley.   1 quart cold water.

Wash barley, add water, and let soak four hours. Cook in same water until water is reduced one-half, if it is to be used for infant feeding; for adults reduce to one cup. Salt and cream may be added, or lemon juice and sugar, as the case may require.

### Toast Water.

2 slices stale bread.  1 cup boiling water.

Cut stale bread in one-third inch slices and remove crusts. Put in pan and bake in a slow oven until thoroughly dried and well browned. Break in small pieces, add water, cover, let stand one hour. Squeeze through cheese cloth. Season with salt, and serve hot or cold. It often proves efficient in extreme cases of nausea.

### Albumen Water. 14 Calories.

White 1 egg.  ½ cup cold water.

Stir white of egg with silver fork to set free the albumen, that it may easily dissolve, as water is added gradually. Strain and serve. A few grains salt may be added if liked.

### Albumen Water with Beef Extract. 14 Calories.

White 1 egg.  ¼ cup boiling water.
¼ teaspoon Liebeg's Beef Extract.  Few grains salt.
Few grains celery salt.

Dissolve beef extract in boiling water. Stir white of egg, using silver fork; then pour on gradually, while stirring constantly, hot mixture. Season with salt and celery salt.

### Apple Water.

1 large sour apple.  ½ cup boiling water.
Sugar.  Lemon juice.

Wipe and core apple. Fill cavity with sugar. Bake in small china dish with enough water to prevent burning. When soft, mash, add boiling water, and let stand twenty minutes. Strain through cheese cloth and add lemon juice to taste.

### Syrup for Fruit Beverages.

¾ cup sugar. ¾ cup boiling water.

Add sugar to boiling water, and place on front of range. Stir until sugar is dissolved, then let boil, without stirring, twelve minutes. Cool, and bottle.

### Currant Jelly Water I.

2 tablespoons currant jelly. ½ cup cold water.
Lemon juice.

Beat jelly before measuring, add water, gradually, and lemon juice to taste. Strain and serve.

Barberry or crab-apple jelly may be used in place of currant jelly if desired.

### Currant Jelly Water II.

2 tablespoons currant juice. 2 tablespoons lemon juice.
2 tablespoons syrup. ⅔ cup cold water.

Mix ingredients in order given.

### Grape Juice.

2 cups Concord grapes. 1 cup cold water.
⅔ cup sugar.

Wash grapes, pick over, and remove stems. Add water, and cook in a double boiler one and one-fourth hours. Add sugar and cook thirty minutes. Strain through double thickness of cheese cloth, and bottle. For serving, dilute with crushed ice or cold water.

### Raspberry Shrub.

3 quarts raspberries. 1 pint cider vinegar.
Cut sugar.

Pick over raspberries, put one-half in earthen jar, add vinegar, cover, and let stand twenty-four hours. Strain through double thickness cheese cloth. Pour liquor over remaining raspberries, and let stand twenty-four hours.

Again strain liquor through double thickness cheese cloth. To each cup juice add one-half pound sugar. Heat gradually until sugar is dissolved, then let boil twenty minutes. Bottle, and cork. Dilute with water for serving.

### Lemonade.

1½ tablespoons syrup.   2 tablespoons lemon juice.
¾ cup cold water.

Mix syrup and lemon juice and add cold water. Use a glass lemon squeezer or wooden drill for expressing juice, to avoid extracting oil from rind, and strain juice before using.

### Hot Lemonade.

Make same as Lemonade, substituting boiling water in place of cold water.

### Soda or Apollinaris Lemonade.

Make same as Lemonade, substituting soda water or Apollinaris in place of cold water. Syphons of soda may be bought of any druggist or first-class grocer. If kept on the ice it is ready for use when needed.

### Lemonade with Lactose.

3 tablespoons lactose.   2 tablespoons lemon juice.
⅓ cup boiling water.   ¼ cup crushed ice.

Lactose, being less sweet to the taste and equal in food value to cane sugar, may be used in place of the latter to sweeten lemonade, thus increasing its nutritive value. Dissolve lactose in boiling water, cool, and add to fruit juice and crushed ice.

### Egg Lemonade.   120 Calories.

1 egg.   2 tablespoons lemon juice.
1 tablespoon powdered sugar.   2 teaspoons sherry.
¼ cup cold water.   2 tablespoons crushed ice.

Beat egg slightly, add sugar, water, lemon juice, and wine, then strain over crushed ice. Wine may be omitted.

# BEVERAGES.

### Egg Lemonade, with Lactose.

1 egg.
3 tablespoons lactose.
¼ cup boiling water.
2 tablespoons lemon juice.
2 teaspoons sherry or port.
¼ cup crushed ice.

Beat egg slightly; dissolve lactose in boiling water, cool, then add to egg with lemon juice and wine. Strain over crushed ice.

### Irish Moss Lemonade.

¼ cup Irish Moss.
1½ cups cold water.
Lemon juice.
Syrup.

Soak Irish Moss in cold water to cover; drain, and pick over. Put in double boiler with one and one-half cups cold water; cook thirty minutes, and strain.

To one-half cup liquid add lemon juice and syrup to taste. Reheat and serve.

### Irish Moss Jelly.

⅓ cup Irish Moss.
1 cup water.
Lemon juice.
Syrup.

Make same as Irish Moss Lemonade, cooking forty-five minutes. Cool, and serve with a spoon.

Irish Moss Lemonade and Irish Moss Jelly are soothing for throat and lung troubles, and will frequently allay an irritating cough.

### Flaxseed Lemonade.

2 tablespoons flaxseed.
2 cups boiling water.
2 tablespoons lemon juice.
Syrup.

Pick over and wash flaxseed. Cover with boiling water and let simmer one hour. Strain, add lemon juice and syrup. Serve hot or cold. Flaxseed Lemonade is especially desirable in kidney troubles. It proves a soothing drink to the throat and bronchial tubes.

### Flaxseed Tea.

2 tablespoons flaxseed.  1½ tablespoons cream of tartar.
1 quart boiling water.  Syrup.
Slices of lemon.

Pick over and wash flaxseed. Add boiling water and cream of tartar, and let simmer until liquid is reduced one-half. Strain, cool, sweeten, and serve with thinly cut slices of lemon. Kidney trouble is accompanied by fever, and cream of tartar is given to cool the blood.

### Orangeade.

Juice 1 orange.  3 tablespoons finely crushed ice.

Put ice in glass and pour over orange juice. Add syrup to sweeten, if necessary.

### Orange Albumen.

White 1 egg.  2 tablespoons crushed ice.
⅓ cup orange juice.  Syrup.

Stir white of egg, using silver fork, add, gradually, orange juice, and strain over crushed ice; then add syrup if necessary.

### Sherry Albumen. 50 Calories.

White 1 egg.  ½ tablespoon powdered sugar.
1 tablespoon sherry.  2 tablespoons crushed ice.

Beat white of egg until stiff, using egg-beater. Add sherry and sugar, gradually, and continue the beating. Pour over crushed ice and serve with a spoon. Port or Madeira wine may be used in place of sherry.

### Lemon Whey.

¼ cup milk.  2 teaspoons lemon juice.

Add lemon juice to milk and let stand five minutes. Strain through double thickness of cheese cloth.

## BEVERAGES.

### Wine Whey.

¼ cup milk.   3 tablespoons sherry.

Scald milk, add wine, and let stand five minutes. Strain through double thickness of cheese cloth and serve hot or cold.

### Junket Whey.

¾ cup milk.   ¼ Junket tablet, or
1 teaspoon cold water.   1 teaspoon Liquid Rennet.

Heat milk until luke warm, add tablet or rennet dissolved in cold water. Let stand in warm place until set, then stir, using silver spoon until thoroughly separated. Strain through double thickness of cheese cloth.

### Clam Water.

1 doz. clams.   2 tablespoons cold water.

Wash clams and scrub with a brush, changing the water several times. Put in saucepan, add water, cover, and cook until shells open. Remove clams from shell, adding liquor which comes from them to liquor already in saucepan. Strain liquor through double thickness of cheese cloth. Serve hot, cold, or frozen.

### Oyster Liquor.

½ pt. oysters.   ⅓ cup cold water.

Chop oysters, add water, heat gradually to boiling point, and let simmer eight minutes. Strain through double thickness cheese cloth.

### Peptonized Milk (Cold Process).

Fairchild's Peptonizing Powder,   ½ cup cold water.
1 tube.   1 pint fresh milk.

Put powder into a sterilized quart bottle, add water, and shake until powder is dissolved; then add milk, cover, shake, and place on ice. Use as needed, always returning remainder to ice at once. If ice is not at hand, make enough for but one serving, for if allowed to stand, artificial digestion will go on to such an extent that the milk will have a bitter flavor.

### Peptonized Milk (Warm Process).

Make same as Peptonized Milk (Cold Process); put bottle in vessel of water (115° F.) and keep at same temperature ten minutes. Serve immediately. Put remainder on ice, or bring quickly to boiling point. In either case artificial digestion is checked.

### Hydrochloric Milk.

1 quart milk. 1 pint water.
25 drops dilute Hydrochloric Acid. ( 10 % solution.)

Add milk to water and heat to boiling point; then add Hydrochloric Acid. Cool before serving. Hydrochloric milk has been successfully used in typhoid.

### Albumenized Milk. 99 Calories.

White 1 egg. ½ cup milk.
Few grains salt.

Stir egg, using a silver fork, thus rupturing the cell walls of albuminin, setting free the albumen. Add milk, gradually, and salt, while stirring constantly. Strain and serve. A milk shaker may be used.

### Koumiss.

1 qt. milk. ¼ yeast cake.
1½ tablespoons sugar. 1 tablespoon luke-warm water.

Heat milk to 75° F., add sugar, and yeast cake dissolved in luke-warm water. Fill sterilized beer bottles to within one and one-half inches of top. Cork and shake. Place bottles, inverted, where they can remain at a temperature of 70° F. for ten hours; then put in ice box or cold place, and stand forty-eight hours, shaking occasionally to prevent cream from clogging mouth of bottle. Koumiss is often retained by those suffering from severe gastric trouble and gives variety for fever patients.

### Milk Punch. 188 Calories.

⅔ cup cold milk.  
½ tablespoon sugar.  
Few grains salt.  
1 tablespoon rum, brandy, or whiskey.

Put ingredients in glass, cover with shaker, invert, and shake until frothy. Turn in glass for serving.

### Milk and Ginger Ale.

Mix cold milk and ginger ale in equal parts, and serve at once.

### Ginger Tea.

1 tablespoon molasses.  
½ teaspoon ginger.  
½ cup boiling water.  
½ cup milk.

Mix molasses and ginger, add boiling water gradually, and let boil one minute; then add milk. Serve as soon as thoroughly heated.

### Egg-Nog I. 228 to 250 Calories.

1 egg.  
¾ tablespoon sugar.  
Few grains salt.  
1½ tablespoons sherry, or  
1 tablespoon brandy or rum.  
⅔ cup cold milk.

Beat egg slightly, add sugar, salt, and, slowly, liquor; then add, gradually, milk. Strain and serve.

### Egg-Nog II.

Yolk 1 egg.  
¾ tablespoon sugar.  
Few grains salt.  
White 1 egg.  
1½ tablespoons sherry, or  
1 tablespoon brandy or rum.  
⅔ cup cold milk.

Beat yolk of egg slightly, add sugar, salt, and, slowly, liquor; then add, gradually, milk. Strain and add white of egg beaten stiff.

### Hot Water Egg-Nog. 115 to 137 Calories.

| | |
|---|---|
| 1 egg. | 1 tablespoon sherry, or |
| ¾ tablespoon sugar. | ½ tablespoon brandy. |
| Few grains salt. | ½ cup hot water. |

Beat egg slightly, add sugar, salt, and wine or brandy; then add water gradually, while stirring constantly. To make more palatable set in a pan of hot water and continue stirring until hot enough to be pleasant to the taste, care being taken to keep mixture below the point at which albumen coagulates.

### Coffee Egg-Nog.

| | |
|---|---|
| 1 egg. | Few grains salt. |
| 1 teaspoon sugar. | ⅔ cup filtered coffee. |

Beat egg slightly, add sugar, salt, and coffee gradually, while stirring constantly; then proceed as in Hot Water Egg-Nog. The egg may be beaten until light if a frothy mixture is preferred.

### Pineapple Egg-Nog.

| | |
|---|---|
| 1 egg. | ¼ cup finely crushed ice. |
| 2 tablespoons cold water. | Syrup. |

2 tablespoons juice expressed from fresh pineapple.

Beat egg slightly, add water and fruit juice; strain over crushed ice and sweeten to taste. Pineapple contains a ferment which digests proteids.

### Moxie with Egg.

| | |
|---|---|
| 1 egg. | ½ cup chilled **Moxie**. |

Beat egg slightly, using a wire whisk. Add Moxie and continue the beating.

BEVERAGES. 77

### Egg with Brandy. 180 Calories.

Yolk 1 egg.  
White 1 egg.  
1 tablespoon brandy.  
1 tablespoon powdered sugar.  
Few grains salt.

Beat yolk of egg until thick and lemon color. Beat white of egg until stiff, using a fork; add sugar gradually, continuing the beating, then add beaten yolk, salt, and brandy. Serve in a small glass and eat with a spoon.

### A Cup of Tea.

1 teaspoon tea.  $\frac{3}{4}$ cup freshly boiling water.

Heat a cup, put in tea, pour on water, cover, and let stand in warm place from three to five minutes. Strain into a hot cup, and serve with sugar and cream or milk.

### A Cup of Tea (made with Tea Ball).

1 teaspoon tea  $\frac{1}{2}$ cup freshly boiling water.

Heat cup, and pour in boiling water. Put tea in tea ball, lower into cup, let stand one minute, then remove. Serve with sugar and cream.

### Iced Tea.

$1\frac{1}{2}$ teaspoons tea.  $\frac{1}{2}$ cup freshly boiling water.  
Glass $\frac{1}{2}$ full crushed ice.

Make same as A Cup of Tea, and strain over crushed ice. Serve with a slice or section of lemon, and sugar.

### Russian Tea.

Follow recipe for A Cup of Tea. Serve hot or cold with sugar and a thin slice of lemon, or a few drops of lemon juice.

### Iced Tea with Mint.

Serve Iced Tea with two or three bruised mint leaves.

### A Pot of Tea.

3 teaspoons tea.   2 cups freshly boiling water.

Scald an earthen or china teapot. Put in tea, pour on water and let stand five minutes on back of range. Strain, and serve immediately.

### A Cup of Coffee (filtered).

2 tablespoons coffee,   1 cup freshly boiling
  finely ground.     water.

Scald a coffee pot for making filtered coffee. Put in coffee, pour over water and let stand in warm place until water filters through. If preferred stronger, re-filter. Serve with sugar and cream, scalded milk, or condensed milk.

### Filtered Coffee.

1 tablespoon coffee,   3 tablespoons freshly
  finely ground.     boiling water.

Take a circular piece of thick filter paper six inches in diameter and form into cornucopia shape by folding four times. Place over a hot cup, put in coffee, pour over water, and allow it to filter through. This is a useful way of making coffee when a small quantity is needed in case of an emergency.

### A Pot of Coffee (boiled).

½ cup ground coffee.   ¾ cup cold water.
½ egg.   3 cups freshly boiling water.

Scald a granite-ware coffee pot. Wash egg, break, and beat slightly. Dilute one-half egg with one-half cup cold water, add one-half the crushed shell, and mix with coffee. Turn into coffee pot, pour on boiling water, and stir thoroughly. Let boil three minutes, stir, and pour some into a cup to be sure that spout is free from grounds. Return to coffee pot, pour in remaining cold water, and let stand on back of range ten minutes. The spout of a coffee pot should be covered to prevent escape of aroma. If there is no cap to coffee pot, stuff with soft paper or a piece of cheese cloth. The size of coffee pot should correspond with the quantity of coffee to be made, if the best results are to be secured.

To serve coffee: Put sugar in cup, add cream, and pour on coffee. The flavor is quite different and not satisfactory to the coffee drinker if the coffee is poured into the cup and the sugar and cream passed.

### Black Coffee.

Follow recipe for Filtered Coffee I. or Boiled Coffee, using one-half the quantity of water. Serve without cream, and generally without sugar.

### Cereal Coffee.

1 tablespoon cereal coffee.     1 cup boiling water.
1 tablespoon cold water.

Add coffee to water. Cover, and let boil from eight to ten minutes. Add cold water, and let stand two minutes to settle. Serve with cream and cut sugar.

### Cocoa Shells.

⅓ cup cocoa shells.     2 cups boiling water.

Boil shells and water two hours. As water boils away it will be necessary to add more. Strain, and serve with an equal quantity of hot milk, and sugar.

### Cracked Cocoa.

½ cup cracked cocoa.     2 quarts boiling water.

Boil cracked cocoa and water two hours. As water boils away it will be necessary to add more. Strain, and serve with milk or cream, and sugar.

### Cocoa Shells and Cracked Cocoa.

Follow recipe for Cocoa Shells, adding two tablespoons cracked cocoa. Strain, and serve with milk or cream and sugar.

### Breakfast Cocoa I.  127 Calories.

| | |
|---|---|
| 1 teaspoon breakfast cocoa. | $\frac{1}{3}$ cup boiling water. |
| 1½ teaspoon sugar. | ½ cup scalded milk. |
| Few grains salt. | |

Mix cocoa, sugar, and salt, and add water, gradually, while stirring constantly. Bring to boiling point and let boil one minute. Turn into scalded milk and beat one minute, using a Dover Egg Beater. This is known as milling, and prevents the forming of scum, which is so unsightly.

### Breakfast Cocoa II.

| | |
|---|---|
| 1½ teaspoons breakfast cocoa. | 2 tablespoons boiling water. |
| 1½ teaspoons sugar. | $\frac{2}{3}$ cup milk. |
| Few grains salt. | |

Make same as Breakfast Cocoa I.

### Breakfast Cocoa with Egg.  220 Calories.

Make Breakfast Cocoa II. Break one egg and turn into a silver pitcher. Beat until light and frothy, using a wire whisk. Add cocoa, gradually, and continue the beating. A silver pitcher is used, because the drink keeps its heat, and does not require reheating after being added to the egg.

### Brandy Cocoa.

| | |
|---|---|
| 1½ teaspoons breakfast cocoa. | 3 tablespoons boiling water. |
| 1½ teaspoons sugar. | $\frac{2}{3}$ cup scalded milk. |
| Few grains salt. | 3 teaspoons brandy. |

Make same as Breakfast Cocoa I., adding brandy at the last.

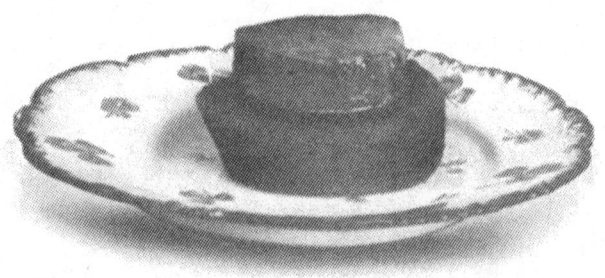

BROILED TENDERLOIN OF BEEF WITH BEEF MARROW
See p. 149

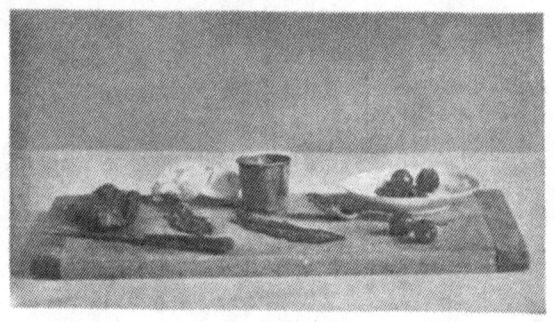

BEEF CUT IN STRIPS FOR SCRAPING. TO BE USED
FOR BEEF BALLS AND SANDWICHES
See p. 141

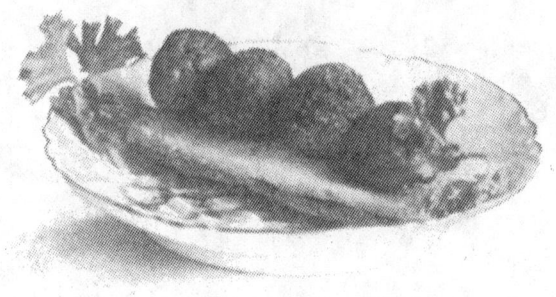

BEEF BALLS
See p. 141

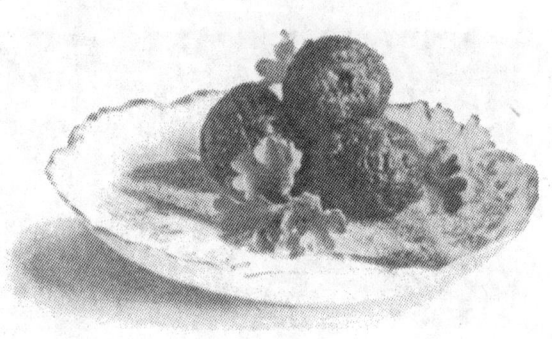

BEEF BALLS
See p. 141

### Cocoa Cordial.

1 teaspoon breakfast cocoa.   ½ cup boiling water.
1 teaspoon sugar.             1½ tablespoons port.
         Few grains salt.

Mix cocoa, sugar, and salt, and add water gradually, while stirring constantly. Boil one minute and add wine.

### Chocolate.

¼ sq. Baker's Chocolate.   ¼ cup boiling water.
1 tablespoon sugar.        ¾ cup scalded milk.
         Few grains salt.

Melt chocolate in small saucepan placed over hot water; then add sugar and salt. Add water gradually, while stirring constantly, and boil one minute. Pour into milk and mill. Serve with or without whipped cream sweetened and flavored with vanilla.

### Egg Cocoa.

White 1 egg.              2 teaspoons cocoa.
2 teaspoons sugar.        ⅔ cup milk.
         Few grains salt.

Beat egg until stiff, add gradually, sugar, salt and cocoa. Add one half of the egg mixture to the milk, turn in a glass and put remaining egg on top.

## CHAPTER XIII.

### GRUELS, BEEF EXTRACTS, AND BEEF TEAS.

GRUELS are cooked mixtures of cereal products and water, or milk and water. In preparing gruels the rules for the cooking of all starchy foods should be observed. Milk or cream, when used in the making of a gruel, should be added just before serving, as milk subjected to a high temperature for a long time is rendered more difficult of digestion. Most patients object to sweetened gruels, therefore avoid the use of sugar in their preparation. In exceptional cases, where it is called for, it may be used sparingly. Gruel should be well seasoned, served hot, and of such a consistency as to be taken through a syphon.

Among gruels, Indian and oat meal take first rank as regards nutritive value. They are heat-producing and slightly laxative. Oatmeal gruel is frequently taken by nursing women to increase the milk supply. It is somewhat more nutritious than an equal quantity of milk; besides, it has the advantage of offering variety to the diet in the form of liquid food. Indian meal gruel is often enjoyed by the aged and the consumptive. Barley gruel acts as an astringent; as do Thickened Milk and Cracker Gruel.

Many preparations are on the market to use in the making of gruels, composed largely of dextrinized starch, malted barley, or evaporated milk. They have largely taken the place of the old-fashioned gruels, for, having been previously cooked, but a short time is required for their preparation. When malt is introduced it assists in the digestion of starch. When economy is considered, their use should be avoided, as they are expensive.

## GRUELS, BEEF EXTRACTS, AND BEEF TEAS.

Beef extract is the expressed juices of beef. Beef tea is the expressed juices of beef diluted with water. Both are composed of water, fat, mineral matter, albuminous juices, and extractives (which give color and flavor). Extractives include creatin, creatinin, and allied compounds (sometimes called meat bases), which closely resemble the thein in tea and the caffein in coffee and have a similar effect upon the nervous system. It is to these compounds that the value of beef extract and beef tea is largely attributable. While they contain a small amount of soluble albumen, the food value is so slight, they must be considered as stimulants rather than nutrients.

Beef tea may be used to advantage.
1. To give variety to a liquid diet.
2. When much water is to be ingested.
3. On account of the warmth that it gives.
4. In cases of weakened digestion.

It stimulates appetite.

Meat extractives are the greatest known stimulants to gastric juice.

Beef extract, being concentrated, may be retained often, if taken in small quantities at frequent intervals, where beef tea could not be borne; on the other hand, beef tea may be taken in larger quantities with satisfying effects, where beef extract would prove insufficient.

Many preparations made from beef are on the market in the form of liquids, powders, meals, or pastes. To some of these a considerable amount of fat is added, which increases their nutritive value; still others are useful only for the flavor and color they impart, and would find better place in the kitchen to be used in the making of soups and sauces than in the sick-room.

Home-made beef tea, if carefully prepared, is usually liked better by a patient, costs much less, and, as a rule, is more nutritious than the manufactured article. It will keep without decomposition, however, but a short time.

Physicians frequently order the preparations on the market, to give variety, and to try, if possible, to please the patient. Again, if home-made beef tea is ordered he is in doubt as to the way in which it will be made, while the manufactured product is uniformly constant.

It is never safe to resort to beef tea as the principal article of diet for more than a few days, as it would mean slow starvation to the patient. Milk, egg, cracker, or bread is added, frequently, to beef extract or beef tea to increase their food value.

Beef, for the making of beef extract and beef tea, should be cut from the upper or lower part of the round of a heavy corn-fed steer. This insures good flavor and a large quantity of juice. One-half pound of such beef will yield two ounces (four tablespoons) of juice, making the price about five cents per ounce. The juice from the lower part of the round is quite as satisfactory and less expensive than that from the upper part.

Beef extract may be served in a colored glass or small china cup. In this way the color, which is objectionable to many, may be concealed.

### Cracker Gruel. 158 Calories.

1 tablespoon rolled and sifted cracker.     ¾ cup milk.
⅛ teaspoon salt.

Scald milk, add cracker, and cook over hot water five minutes, then add salt.

### Dextrinized Cracker Gruel.

1¼ tablespoon browned cracker     ¾ cup milk.
(rolled and sifted).     ⅛ teaspoon salt.

Follow directions for Cracker Gruel. The cracker may be dextrinized by baking for a long time in a very slow oven.

### Rice Gruel.

1 tablespoon rice.     1 cup milk.

Wash rice, cover with cold water, and let stand two hours; drain, add milk to rice, and cook one and one-half hours in top of double boiler. Strain twice through a fine strainer, season with salt. Serve hot or cold.

## GRUELS, BEEF EXTRACTS, AND BEEF TEAS.

### Thickened Milk. 196 Calories.

1 tablespoon flour.          1 cup milk.
Few grains salt.

Scald milk, reserving two tablespoons. Add cold milk, gradually, to flour while stirring constantly to make a smooth paste. Pour into scalded milk, and stir until mixture thickens, then cover, and cook over hot water twenty minutes. Season with salt. An inch piece of stick cinnamon may be cooked with the milk if liked, and tends to reduce a laxative condition. Thickened milk is often given in bowel troubles.

### Barley Gruel I.

1 tablespoon barley flour.     1 cup boiling water.
2 tablespoons cold water.      ½ cup milk.
¼ teaspoon salt.

Add cold water slowly to barley flour to form a thin paste, then add gradually to boiling water, while stirring constantly; let boil fifteen minutes. Add milk, bring to boiling point, season, and strain.

### Barley Gruel II.

1 tablespoon barley flour.     1 cup scalded milk.
2 tablespoons cold milk.      ¼ teaspoon salt.

Add cold milk, slowly, to barley flour to form a thin paste. Add gradually to scalded milk, while stirring constantly. Cook in double boiler twenty minutes. Season, and strain.

### Farina Gruel. 161 Calories.

½ tablespoon farina.      ½ cup milk.
¾ cup boiling water.      1 egg yolk.
¼ teaspoon salt.

Add farina, slowly, to boiling water, while stirring constantly, then let boil twenty minutes. Add milk and reheat. Beat egg yolk slightly, dilute with two tablespoons mixture, add to remaining mixture, season, and strain.

### Indian Meal Gruel.

1 tablespoon granulated Indian meal.
½ tablespoon flour.
¼ teaspoon salt.
3 tablespoons cold water.
2 cups boiling water.
Milk or cream.

Mix meal, flour, and salt. Add cold water slowly to form a thin paste, then add gradually to boiling water, while stirring constantly, and let boil one hour. Add milk or cream to meet the needs of the patient.

### Oatmeal Gruel I.

¼ cup rolled oats.
1½ cups boiling water.
¼ teaspoon salt.
Milk or cream.

Add oats mixed with salt to boiling water, let boil two minutes, then cook over hot water one hour. Strain, bring to boiling point, and add milk or cream to meet the needs of the case.

### Oatmeal Gruel II.

⅓ cup coarse oatmeal.
1½ cups cold water.
½ teaspoon salt.
Milk or cream.

Pound oatmeal in a mortar, or roll until mealy. Put in tumbler, add one-third of the water, while stirring constantly, let settle, and pour off mealy water. Repeat twice, using remaining water. Boil mealy water thirty minutes, then add salt, milk, or cream. This gives a starchy gruel, delicate in flavor, but not as nutritious as Oatmeal Gruel I.

### Beef Extract.

½ lb. beefsteak, from round, cut one inch thick.
Salt.

Remove fat and wipe steak with a cloth wrung out of cold water. Place on heated wire broiler, and broil four minutes, turning every ten seconds for the first minute (to prevent the escape of juices), then occasionally. Remove from broiler to warm plate and cut in pieces of correct size to fit meat press or metal lemon-squeezer. Make several gashes in pieces on both sides, put in press or lemon-squeezer, and express juice. Turn juice into cup set in saucepan of hot water. Season with salt, and serve at once. Care must be taken that cup does not become sufficiently hot to coagulate albuminous juices.

### Beef Extract with Port.

Serve cold Beef Extract, flavored with port.

### Frozen Beef Extract.

Freeze Beef Extract.

### Beef Tea I.

Dilute Beef Extract with an equal quantity of hot water.

### Beef Tea II.

| | |
|---|---|
| 1 lb. beefsteak, cut from round. | 2 cups cold water. Salt. |

Remove fat, wipe and cut beef in small pieces or put through meat chopper. Put in canning jar, add cold water, cover, and let stand twenty minutes. Place on trivet in kettle of cold water, having water surround jar as high as contents. Heat water gradually, keeping temperature at 130° F. for two hours, then increase temperature slightly until the liquid becomes a chocolate color and the albuminous juices are slightly coagulated; otherwise the beef tea will have a raw taste. Strain, season and serve.

### Beef Tea III.

Follow recipe for Beef Tea II. Put beef in top of double boiler, add cold water and a two-and-one-half inch cube of ice. Have cold water in under part of double boiler, cover and let stand twenty minutes. Place on range, heat slowly, and keep water just below boiling point for two hours. Strain, season and serve.

## CHAPTER XIV.

### BREAD.

BREAD may be called, without error of statement, "the staff of life," inasmuch as it is used by all civilized peoples as their staple article of food, and furnishes proteid, carbohydrate, mineral matter, and a small quantity of fat. The deficiency in fat is usually supplied by spreading bread with butter.

Breads may be considered under two great classes: —

1. Fermented,
    Made light by the use of a ferment, yeast usually being employed.
2. Unfermented,
    Made light by the use of soda and cream of tartar, or baking powder.

In either case the lightness is due to the development of carbon dioxid ($CO_2$). In the first instance this change is brought about during the process of fermentation. There are various kinds of fermentation, each of which is caused by special organisms. The organisms found in the yeast plant are the ones which apply to bread making. They have the power of changing starch to sugar, and sugar to alcohol and carbon dioxid. In the second case the change is brought about by chemical reaction. By the action of moisture and heat, the gas in the bicarbonate of soda is liberated by the acid in the cream of tartar.

The necessary ingredients for a loaf of bread are flour, water, and yeast. To these may be added shortening, salt, sugar, and milk.

Bread made with water, flour, salt, and yeast keeps fresh longer, and is less liable to sour, than when milk is used for the wetting, but is of a tougher consistency, and not as palatable. When shortening is added with either milk or water the bread is tenderer and better tasting. The addition of a little sugar — one tablespoon to six cups of flour — hastens the rising, and has no appreciable effect on the taste. The United States Department of Agriculture, Farmer's Bulletin 112, recommends the use of milk for bread making, as it adds to the proteid as well as the fuel value of the loaf.

Hard spring wheat flour is the best adapted to bread making, as it contains gluten in the right proportion to produce the spongy loaf. Gluten is the chief proteid of wheat. Its elastic, tenacious qualities, when mixed with water and acted upon by yeast, allow the gas formed to expand without danger of escape, making light the entire mass. The strength of a flour is determined largely by the quantity of gluten it contains. The larger the quantity of gluten, the more water it will take up, and the greater the yield in number of loaves to the barrel.

Entire wheat, Graham, and white flour are all products of wheat. Entire wheat flour may be bought either fine or coarse. Graham flour is a dark flour product containing a perceptible quantity of the coarse inner bran coats of the wheat.

Rye flour ranks next to wheat flour for bread making purposes. It is of darker color, and its gluten is less elastic and tenacious. In making rye bread it is desirable to use white flour in combination with rye flour.

Oats and barley are seldom used in the making of bread. Their gluten is even less tenacious than that of rye. From corn meal it is impossible to make a raised loaf, for none of its proteid is in the form of gluten.

### Composition and Food Value of Standard Flours.

| Kind. | Proteid. | Carbohydrate. | Fat. | Mineral matter. | Calories per pound |
|---|---|---|---|---|---|
| White | 11.4% | 75.1% | 1.0% | 0.5% | 1635 |
| Entire wheat | 13.8% | 71.9% | 1.9% | 1.0% | 1650 |
| Graham flour | 13.3% | 71.4% | 2.2% | 1.8% | 1645 |
| Rye flour | 6.8% | 78.7% | 0.9% | 0.7% | 1620 |

From this table it may be seen that there is no appreciable difference between the fuel value of bread, whether made from white or entire wheat flour. Bread made from Graham flour contains so much of the bran coats of the wheat that it is forced through the digestive tract so quickly that absorption is less complete, and the system gets less nutritive value from it than from other breads. Nevertheless, there are times when its use is to be recommended. If the intestines do their work slowly and incompletely, it acts as a stimulus to peristalsis.

### Yeast.

Yeast is a minute single-celled plant of fungus growth which reproduces itself in two ways: —

1. By sending out buds which break off as new plants.
2. By forming spores which develop into new plants, under favorable conditions.

Conditions most favorable for its growth: —

1. Warmth (78° F.).
2. Moisture.
3. Sugar or starch converted into sugar.
4. Nitrogenous soil.
5. Oxygen.

The most favorable temperature for the growth of the yeast plant is 78° F. Yeast is killed at a moist heat of 140° F. or a dry heat of 212° F. Yeast will survive freezing temperature (32° F.), and if again placed under favorable conditions will grow and thrive.

While the yeast plant is active when well furnished with air, it is capable of obtaining a supply of oxygen by splitting up sugar and starch.

In bread making the side products of fermentation are almost as important as the carbon dioxid and alcohol, as they give flavor and aroma to the products.

Wild yeast plants are found floating in the air, and it is by the cultivation of these that pure yeast cultures are obtained. Standard brands of compressed yeast cakes are most satisfactory for bread making and are almost universally used. They contain a larger number of yeast plants to a given bulk than any other form of yeast, either liquid or dry.

Yeast cakes should be used only when fresh, and while they keep fresh but a few days, there is seldon difficulty in obtaining a satisfactory supply. A fresh yeast cake is known by its light color, and absence from dark streaks.

### Bread Making.

Fermented bread is made by mixing to a dough flour, with a liquid (water, milk, or milk and water), salt, and a ferment (yeast), sugar being usually added to hasten fermentation. The dough is then kneaded until smooth, elastic to the touch, and bubbles may be seen on the surface, to thoroughly mix the ingredients, to distribute uniformly the yeast, and to incorporate air; then covered for rising, and allowed to remain at a temperature of 69° to 78° F. until it doubles its bulk. During this time the yeast has produced a ferment which changes some of the starch to sugar, and the sugar in turn to alcohol and carbon dioxid. Still another ferment appears which peptonizes some of the gluten of the wheat.

It is then cut down, and again kneaded, to break bubbles and distribute evenly the gas already formed. If allowed to rise too long the result will be a sour bread. If it is not convenient to shape the dough when it has doubled its bulk, it may be cut down, thus checking fermentation for the time being, then set in a cool place to let rise again. This may be done without injury to the finished loaf; in fact many consider the second rising an improvement. Sour bread shows either lack of the knowledge of bread making or carelessness.

Where bread is mixed in the morning, when one is able to keep a watch on it during the entire rising, a uniform temperature is best accomplished by placing bowl containing dough in a larger vessel of water kept at a temperature of 100° F.

After the yeast has done its work (which is accomplished when a certain amount of alcohol is produced) bacterial action begins, which gives rise to acetic, lactic, and butyric fermentation, which are the causes of sour bread. These micro-organisms may enter the mixture through the flour, water, or air, and a few are present in the yeast cake. Salt retards the action of bacteria.

Quick rising, or five-hour bread, requires a larger quantity of yeast cake than bread which is allowed to rise over night, but is generally more satisfactory. There are, however, some who prefer the flavor obtained by the long rising. In the following recipes five-hour bread only will be considered. These recipes may be used where bread is allowed to rise over night if one-fourth yeast cake is allowed to each pint of liquid.

A sponge is a mixture of liquid, flour, and yeast cake of such a consistency to pour or drop from a spoon. Many in making bread prefer first making a sponge, allowing that to rise until light, and then adding flour to knead.

### Shaping Bread Doughs.

Bread dough, properly risen, is ready for shaping into loaves, biscuits, or rolls. Cut off dough the desired size, knead until smooth, avoiding seams underneath, place in buttered pan, cover, again let rise to double its bulk, when it is ready for baking.

Biscuits or rolls may be shaped in a great variety of ways but always see to it that they are made small. Hot fresh raised bread is not a suitable article of diet for the sick and convalescent.

Sometimes stale biscuits or rolls, reheated, may be used, and twice baked bread, in the form of pulled bread and Zwieback, is especially recommended.

### Baking of Bread.

Bread is baked
1. To kill the yeast plant (accomplished at 158° F.).
2. To render the starch soluble.
3. To drive off alcohol and carbon dioxid.
4. To form a dextrinized crust of sweet, pleasant flavor.

It is a common error to bake loaf bread insufficiently. While it requires a hot oven, it should continue to rise for about fifteen minutes after going into the oven, then the rising should cease and the loaf begin to brown.

A loaf of bread of medium size requires from one to one and one-fourth hours for baking.

### Digestibility.

Freshly baked bread cannot be sufficiently masticated to render it easy of digestion. Stale bread, from thirty-six to forty-eight hours old, if thoroughly masticated, is well digested and absorbed.

Butter spread on bread not only increases its nutritive value, but tends to assist its digestibility.

### Water Bread.

2 cups boiling water.
1½ tablespoons butter.
1 tablespoon sugar.
1¼ teaspoons salt.
1 yeast cake (dissolved in ¼ cup lukewarm water).
6 cups sifted flour.

Put butter, sugar, and salt in bowl without a lip. Pour on boiling water, and when lukewarm add dissolved yeast cake and five cups flour, then stir until thoroughly mixed, using a knife or spoon. Add remaining flour, mix, and turn on a floured cloth; knead, return to bowl, and cover with a cloth and board or tin cover. Let rise until mixture has doubled its bulk, cut down, toss on a floured cloth, knead, shape, let rise again, and bake. Remove from pan, place side down on wire rack, that the air may have an opportunity to circulate around it. If a soft crust is desired, cover with a towel. Avoid putting in bread box until thoroughly cooled, as it keeps better, and is less liable to become mouldy. Never wrap bread in a cloth, as the cloth will absorb moisture and transmit an unpleasant taste to the bread.

### Pulled Bread.

Make Water Bread in long loaves, so that the grain of the bread extends the entire length of the loaf. Remove crusts while bread is warm, and pull bread apart in stick-shape pieces of uniform size. Put sticks in pan and bake in a slow oven until thoroughly dried and delicately browned.

### Milk and Water Bread.

1 cup scalded milk.
1 cup boiling water.
1½ tablespoons butter.
1 tablespoon sugar.
1¼ teaspoons salt.
1 yeast cake dissolved in ¼ cup lukewarm water.
6 cups flour.

Make and bake same as Water Bread.

### Entire Wheat Bread I.

1 cup scalded milk
1 cup boiling water.
1½ tablespoons butter.
1¼ teaspoons salt.
1 yeast cake dissolved in ¼ cup lukewarm water.
1 cup white flour.
Entire Wheat flour (enough to knead).
3 tablespoons molasses.

Make same as Water Bread, adding molasses after the first rising.

### Entire Wheat Bread II.

2 cups scalded milk.
1 teaspoon salt
1 yeast cake dissolved in ¼ cup lukewarm water.
3¼ cups Entire Wheat flour (coarse).
2¾ cups white flour.
¼ cup sugar or ⅓ cup molasses.

Add sugar and salt to milk; when lukewarm add dissolved yeast cake and flour. Toss on a floured cloth.

Knead slightly and handle quickly to prevent dough from sticking to cloth and hands. Put in bowl, cover, and let rise. Shape, let rise again, and bake. If molasses is used, add after the first rising.

### Graham Bread.

2½ cups liquid (water or milk and water).
⅓ cup molasses.
1½ teaspoons salt.
1 yeast cake dissolved in ¼ cup lukewarm water.
3 cups Graham flour.
3 cups flour.

Add molasses and salt to liquid, when lukewarm add dissolved yeast cake and flour. Beat thoroughly, cover, and let rise. Again beat, and turn into buttered bread pans, having pans one-half full. Let rise, and bake. Graham bread should not quite double its bulk during the last rising. A satisfactory way of making this bread is to first make a sponge of the white flour and when well risen add molasses and Graham flour.

### Rye Bread.

1 cup scalded milk.
1 cup boiling water.
1½ tablespoons butter.
⅓ cup brown sugar.
1½ teaspoons salt.
1 yeast cake dissolved in ¼ cup lukewarm water.
3 cups flour.
Rye meal (enough to knead).

Add milk and water to shortening, sugar, and salt. When lukewarm add dissolved yeast cake and flour. Beat thoroughly, cover, and let rise, add rye meal until dough is stiff enough to knead. Toss on floured cloth, knead, let rise, shape in loaves, let rise again, and bake.

### Oat Bread.

2 cups boiling water.
1 cup rolled oats.
1 tablespoon butter.
⅓ cup molasses.
½ tablespoon salt.
1 yeast cake dissolved in ½ cup lukewarm water.
4½ cups flour.

Add boiling water to oats and butter and let stand one hour. Then add remaining ingredients, beat thoroughly, and let rise, turn into buttered bread pans, let rise again, and bake in a hot oven.

### Health Food Bread.

| | |
|---|---|
| 1 cup warm wheat mush. | 1 tablespoon butter. |
| ¼ cup brown sugar. | 1 yeast cake dissolved in |
| ½ teaspoon salt. | ¼ cup lukewarm water. |

Flour.

Mix ingredients in the order given, using enough flour to knead. Knead, cover, let rise, shape, put into buttered pan, cover, let rise again, and bake in a hot oven.

### Bread Sticks.

| | |
|---|---|
| 1 cup scalded milk. | 1 yeast cake dissolved in |
| ¼ cup butter. | ¼ cup lukewarm water. |
| 1½ tablespoons sugar. | White 1 egg. |
| ½ teaspoon salt. | 3¾ cups flour. |

Add butter, sugar, and salt to milk; when lukewarm add dissolved yeast cake, white of egg, well beaten, and flour. Knead, cover, let rise, shape, pile on buttered tin sheet, cover, let rise again, and bake. The oven should be hot enough to stop the rising at once, then the heat should be reduced, that sticks may be crisp and dry.

To shape bread sticks, form small biscuits, then roll biscuits, using both hands (on part of board where there is no flour) until of desired length, uniform thickness, and round at ends.

### Bran Muffins.

| | |
|---|---|
| ½ cup flour. | 1 cup bran. |
| ½ teaspoon soda. | ½ cup milk. |
| ¼ teaspoon salt. | 2½ tablespoons molasses. |

1 egg.

Mix and sift flour, soda, and salt. Add bran, molasses, and milk; then egg well beaten. Bake in hot buttered gem pans.

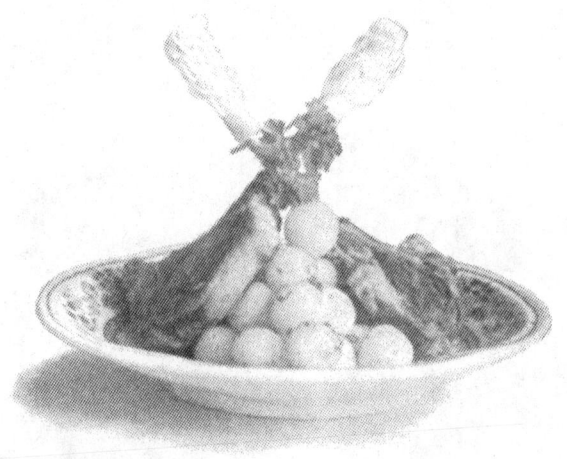

**PAN-BROILED FRENCH CHOPS WITH POTATO BALLS**
See p. 143

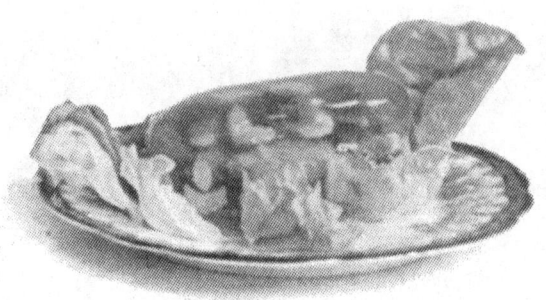

**JELLIED SWEETBREAD**
See p. 144

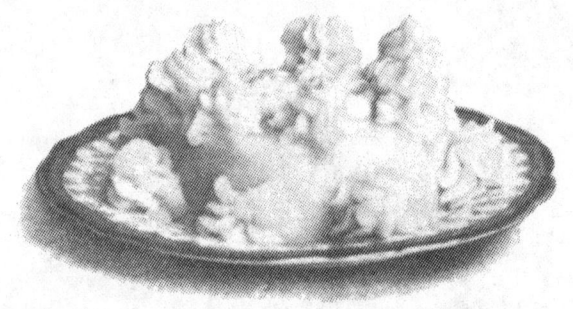

CREAMED CHICKEN IN POTATO BORDER
See p. 146

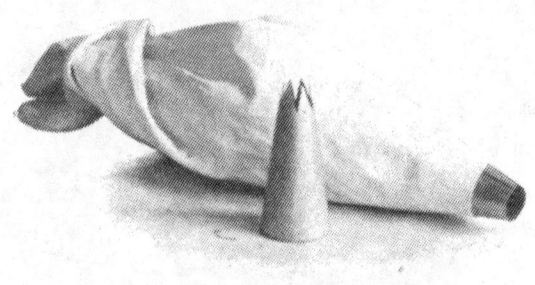

PASTRY BAG AND TUBES

## BREAD.

### Invalid Muffins.

| | |
|---|---|
| 1 cup bread flour. | ½ cup milk. |
| 1 teaspoon baking powder. | Whites 2 eggs. |
| ½ teaspoon salt. | 2 tablespoons melted butter. |

Mix and sift dry ingredients, add milk gradually, eggs well beaten, and melted butter. Bake in moderate oven in buttered gem pans. Let stand in oven, after baking, with door ajar, that crust may be dry and crisp. To be eaten hot or cold.

### White Corn Meal Cake.

¼ cup white corn meal.   ½ cup scalded milk.
½ teaspoon salt.

Add salt to corn meal, and pour on, gradually, milk. Turn into a buttered shallow pan to the depth of one-fourth inch. Bake in a moderate oven until crisp. Split, and spread with butter.

### Rusks (Zwieback).

| | |
|---|---|
| ½ cup milk. | ¼ cup sugar. |
| 2 yeast cakes. | ¼ cup melted butter. |
| ½ teaspoon salt. | 3 eggs. |

Flour.

Scald milk, and when lukewarm, add yeast cakes, and as soon as yeast cakes are dissolved add salt and one cup flour. Cover, and let rise until light; then add sugar, butter, eggs unbeaten, and flour enough to handle. Knead, shape, and place close together in two parallel rows two inches apart on a buttered sheet. Let rise again, and bake in a hot oven twenty-five minutes. When cold cut diagonally in one-half inch slices, and brown in a slow oven.

To shape rusks make small biscuit and roll on part of cloth where there is no flour, using one hand until four and one-half inches long, of uniform size, and round at ends.

### Dry Toast.

Cut stale bread in one-third inch slices and remove crusts. Place in wire toaster, lock toaster, and hold over clear fire to dry one side, holding some distance from coals; turn, and dry other side. Hold nearer to coals and color a golden brown, first on one side, then on other. The moisture in the bread should be nearly evaporated, thus making the toast dry and crisp. By this means of toasting some of the starch becomes dextrinized, and the bread is thus rendered easier of digestion. If only charred on the outside and soft in the inside, it forms in the stomach a soggy, indigestible mass.

Toast should never be piled one slice on another, except it be cut in suitable shapes, that it may be piled log-cabin fashion. If a toast rack is not at hand, balance toast against cup placed in warm plate until serving time.

If toast is desired in finger-shaped pieces, triangles, or fancy shapes, it must be cut as desired before being toasted.

### Water Toast. 180 Calories.

2 slices dry toast.   ¾ teaspoon salt.
1 cup boiling water.  ½ tablespoon butter.

Drop toast, each piece separately, in boiling salted water, remove to hot dish, spread with butter, and serve at once.

### Cracker Toast.

Split and toast common crackers. Spread generously with butter, moisten with salted boiling water, put in hot dish, and pour over scalded milk.

### Milk Toast.

2 slices dry toast.    ¾ cup scalded milk.
¾ tablespoon butter.   ¼ teaspoon salt.

Butter bread, arrange on hot dish, and pour over milk to which salt has been added.

### Sippets with Milk. 242 Calories.

1 slice dry toast.  
½ tablespoon butter.  
¾ cup scalded milk.  
⅛ teaspoon salt.

Cut toast in small pieces of uniform size. Put remaining ingredients in small heated bowl, add toast, and serve at once.

### Dip Toast. 408 Calories.

2 slices dry toast.  
¾ tablespoon butter.  
¼ teaspoon salt.  
1½ tablespoons flour.  
1 cup scalded milk.  
2 tablespoons cold milk.

Add cold milk gradually to flour to make a smooth paste. Turn into scalded milk, stirring constantly at first until mixture thickens. Cook over hot water twenty minutes. Add salt, and butter in small pieces. Dip slices of toast separately in sauce. When soft remove to serving-dish, and pour over remaining sauce.

### Cream Toast. 476 Calories.

2 slices dry toast.  
1 tablespoon flour.  
¾ cup scalded thin cream.  
2 tablespoons cold milk.  
¼ teaspoon salt.

Follow recipe for making Dip Toast.

### Croustades of Bread.

Cut stale bread in two-inch slices, and cut slices in square, circular, or diamond-shaped pieces.

Remove centres, making cases, leaving walls as thin as possible. Brush over with melted butter, and brown in a moderate oven. The top of croustades may be brushed over with slightly beaten white of egg, then dipped in dry, finely chopped parsley. To be filled with creamed vegetables, oysters, or chicken.

## CHAPTER XV.

### BREAKFAST CEREALS.

BREAKFAST cereals are made from oats, corn, wheat, or rice. At the present time so great is the number upon the market, that one has an extensive variety from which to choose. They are put up in one or two pound packages, almost all of them having been partially cooked. Printed directions are given for the cooking, the time for which is always insufficient.

Breakfast cereals are valuable, inexpensive foods, and their daily use is strongly recommended. It is a fact to be regretted that they are not more freely employed by the poorer classes in our own country.

#### Table showing Composition.

| Article. | Proteid. | Fat. | Starch. | Mineral Matter. | Water. | Calorie Value per pound. |
|---|---|---|---|---|---|---|
| Rolled Oats | 16.9% | 7.2% | 66.8% | 1.9% | 7.2% | 1860 |
| Corn Meal | 8.9 | 2.2 | 75.1 | 0.9 | 12.9 | 1655 |
| Hominy | 8.2 | 0.6 | 78.9 | 0.4 | 10.8 | 1645 |
| Wheat Breakfast Cereal | 12.3 | 1.4 | 75.0 | 0.9 | 10.4 | 1685 |
| Rice | 7.8 | 0.4 | 79.0 | 0.4 | 12.4 | 1630 |
| Macaroni | 11.7 | 1.6 | 72.9 | 0.3 | 10.8 | 1640 |

*Bulletin 28, U. S. Department of Agriculture.*

Oat preparations rank first as regards nutritive value. They contain a stimulating principle which is lacking in the other cereals. Owing to the fact that they hold a large amount of fat and cellulose, there are many with whom they disagree. In such cases their use should be avoided. As regards heat-giving properties, corn ranks next to oats, therefore both are especially adapted for a winter diet. They are slightly laxative.

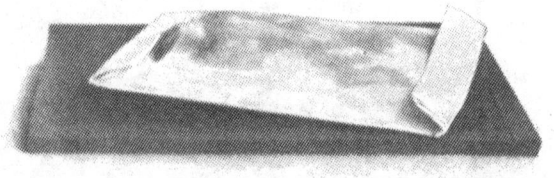

BONED BIRD IN PAPER CASE, READY FOR BROILING
See p. 148

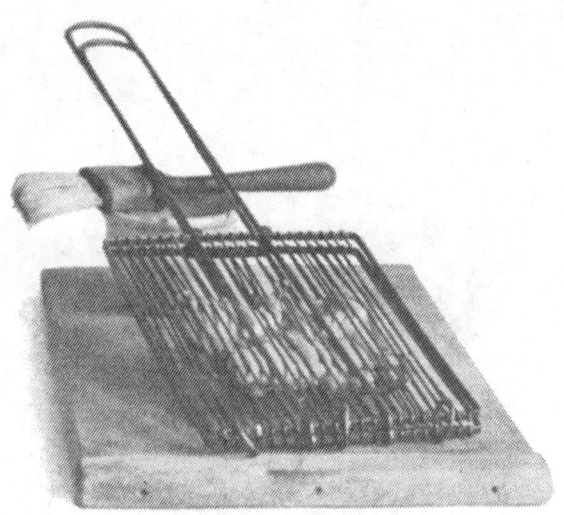

QUAIL SPLIT AND READY FOR BROILING
See p. 148

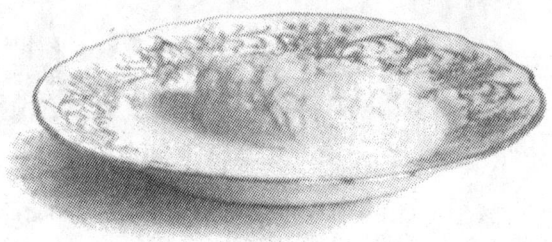

CHICKEN AND RICE CUTLET
See p. 147

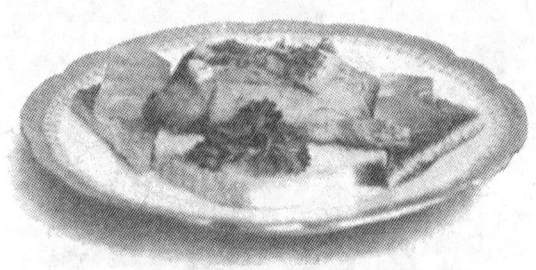

BROILED QUAIL ON TOAST, GARNISHED WITH TOAST
POINTS, CUBES OF JELLY, LEMON, AND PARSLEY
See p. 147

# BREAKFAST CEREALS.

A kernel of wheat is deficient in but one of the five food principles, namely fat, to make it an ideal food. For this reason wheat preparations may be used to advantage throughout the year. It is a fact that wheat is more largely consumed than any other cereal, rice holding second place.

Rice contains more starch and less fat than any of the cereals. It has a delicate flavor, but is not as popular in the United States, except in the southern part, as wheat, oats, or corn.

Macaroni is made from wheat flour rich in proteid, and water. It is manufactured to some extent in this country, but the best brands come from Italy. Like the cereals, it is an inexpensive, nutritive food.

All the cereals contain a large percentage of starch, in consequence of which they should be thoroughly cooked. The following points must be followed for the best results:

1. Double boiler, the utensil for cooking.
2. Correct proportions of water, cereal, and salt.
3. Temperature of water, boiling point (212° F.).
4. Time for cooking.
5. Manner of serving.

In cooking cereals the double boiler employed should correspond in size to the quantity to be prepared. The following recipesc all for the use of the smallest ones put upon the market.

Oftentimes where cereals have not proved popular, it is due to the fact that they have been improperly cooked or have been served with poor milk, rather than with rich milk or thin cream. To avoid monotony, vary the kind of cereal, never allowing the same preparation to appear on consecutive mornings.

### Digestibility.

Breakfast cereals, if properly cooked, are well digested and absorbed, holding close rank to animal foods. Of the proteid there is a loss of fifteen per cent; of the fat, ten per cent; of the carbohydrate, two per cent.

### Table for cooking Cereals.

| Kind. | Quantity. | Water. | Time. |
|---|---|---|---|
| Rolled Oats | $\frac{1}{3}$ cup (1 oz.) | $\frac{7}{8}$ cup | 1 hr. |
| Fould's Wheat Germ | $3\frac{3}{4}$ tablespoons | $\frac{7}{8}$ cup | 45 min. to 1 hr. |
| Wheatena | $3\frac{1}{3}$ tablespoons | 1 cup | 45 min. to 1 hr. |
| Wheatlet | $3\frac{2}{3}$ tablespoons | $\frac{7}{8}$ cup | 45 min. to 1 hr. |
| Toasted Wheat | $3\frac{1}{4}$ tablespoons | $\frac{7}{8}$ cup | 45 min. to 1 hr |
| Vitos | 3 tablespoons | 1 cup | 45 min to 1 hr. |
| Pettijohn | $\frac{1}{2}$ cup (scant) | $\frac{7}{8}$ cup | 30 min. |
| Corn meal | $3\frac{1}{4}$ tablespoons | 1 cup | 3 hrs. |
| Hominy (fine) | $3\frac{1}{2}$ tablespoons | 1 cup | $1\frac{1}{2}$ hrs. |
| Rice | $2\frac{2}{3}$ tablespoons | $\frac{3}{4}$ cup | 45 min. to 1 hr |
| Rolled Rye Flakes | $\frac{1}{3}$ cup | $\frac{3}{4}$ cup | 30 min. |

### Rolled Oats Mush. 256 Calories.

$\frac{1}{3}$ cup rolled oats.　　　　$\frac{3}{4}$ cup boiling water.
$\frac{1}{4}$ teaspoon salt.

Add oats mixed with salt to boiling water gradually, while stirring constantly. Boil two minutes, then steam in double boiler one hour. Serve with one tablespoon sugar and one-fourth cup thin cream.

### Wheatena with Fruit.

$3\frac{1}{3}$ tablespoons Wheatena.　Fresh fruit (sliced peaches,
1 cup boiling water.　　　　　　strawberries, or raspberries,
$\frac{1}{4}$ teaspoon salt.　　　　　　or baked apples).

Follow directions for cooking Rolled Oats Mush. Serve with sugar, cream, and fruit.

### Wheatlet Mush with Fruit.

$3\frac{2}{3}$ tablespoons Wheatlet.　$\frac{1}{4}$ teaspoon salt.
$\frac{7}{8}$ cup boiling water.　　　$\frac{1}{3}$ cup dates, stoned and cut in quarters.

Follow directions for cooking Rolled Oats Mush. Add dates, cook two minutes, and serve with cream.

# BREAKFAST CEREALS. 103

### Wheat Mush with Egg.

To Wheatena or Wheatlet Mush add, just before serving, white one egg beaten stiff. Serve with sugar and cream and fruit when desired.

### Hominy Mush.

3⅛ tablespoons fine hominy.   1 cup boiling water.
¼ teaspoon salt.

Follow directions for cooking Rolled Oats Mush. Cook from one to one and one-half hours. Serve with sugar and cream, or butter and maple syrup.

### Corn Meal Mush.

3⅓ tablespoons granulated corn meal.   ¼ teaspoon salt.
⅓ cup cold water or milk.   ⅔ cup boiling water.

Add water or milk, gradually, to corn meal mixed with salt. Pour into boiling water, placed on front of range, while stirring constantly. Boil two minutes, then steam in double boiler three hours. Serve with butter and maple syrup.

### Oat Jelly. 116 Calories.

⅓ cup rolled oats.   ¼ teaspoon salt.
1½ cups boiling water.

Add oats mixed with salt to boiling water gradually. Boil two minutes, then steam in double boiler forty-five minutes to one hour. Force through a fine strainer, mould, chill, and serve with sugar and cream.

### Boiled Rice.

2¾ tablespoons rice.   2½ cups boiling water.
½ teaspoon salt.

Pick over rice; add slowly to boiling salted water, not checking boiling of water. Let boil twenty-five minutes, or until soft. Old rice absorbs more water than new rice, and takes longer for the cooking. Drain in coarse strainer, and pour over one cup hot water. Return to saucepan, cover, place on back of range, and let stand to dry off, when kernels are distinct. Serve with sugar and cream.

### Steamed Rice.

2¾ tablespoons rice.        ¾ cup water.
¼ teaspoon salt.

Put salt and water in top of double boiler, place on range, and add gradually well-washed rice, stirring with a fork. Boil three minutes, cover, place over under part double boiler, and steam forty-five minutes; uncover, that steam may escape. Serve with sugar and cream. Rice when used as a dessert may be cooked with half milk and half water instead of all water.

How to Wash Rice. Put rice in strainer, place strainer over bowl nearly full of cold water. Rub rice gently between hands, lift strainer from bowl and change water; repeat three or four times, when water will be quite clear.

### Boiled Macaroni. 115 Calories.

Break macaroni in one-inch pieces; there should be one-fourth cup. Cook in two cups boiling salted water, until soft. Turn into strainer, and pour over one pint cold water to prevent pieces from adhering. Return to saucepan, add two tablespoons cream, and re-heat. Season with one-eighth teaspoon salt.

### Macaroni with White Sauce. 228 Calories.

¼ cup macaroni.        ½ tablespoon flour.
½ tablespoon butter.        ½ cup milk.
¼ teaspoon salt.

Cook macaroni as for Boiled Macaroni. Melt butter, add flour, and pour on, gradually, while stirring constantly, the milk. Season with salt, and add macaroni.

### Baked Macaroni.

Butter a baking-dish, fill with Macaroni with White Sauce. Cover with buttered cracker crumbs, and bake until crumbs are brown.

For buttered cracker crumbs allow one tablespoon melted butter to one-fourth cup crumbs.

### Macaroni with Oysters.

Cover bottom of buttered baking-dish with Boiled Macaroni. Cover macaroni with six oysters, dredge generously with flour, and sprinkle with salt and pepper. Dot over with one tablespoon butter, add remaining macaroni, and cover with buttered crumbs. Bake twelve to fifteen minutes in a hot oven.

## CHAPTER XVI.

### EGGS.

AN egg consists of the shell, the membrane which lies next the shell, the white, and the yolk, the yolk being balanced in the white by means of two spiral springs. On the yolk of a fertile egg can be found a spot which is the germ.

#### Composition of Hen's Egg.

|  | Refuse | Water | Protein. | Fat. | Ash. | Fuel value per pound. Calories. |
|---|---|---|---|---|---|---|
| Whole egg as purchased | 11.2% | 65.5% | 11.9% | 9.3% | 0 9% | 635 |
| Whole egg, edible portion | ... | 73 7 | 13 4 | 10.5 | 1.0 | 720 |
| White | ... | 86.2 | 12.3 | 0.2 | 0.6 | 250 |
| Yolk | ... | 49.5 | 15.7 | 33.3 | 1.1 | 1,705 |

*Farmer's Bulletin No.* 128, *U. S. Department of Agriculture.*

Eggs furnish a valuable, concentrated proteid food and are a useful substitute for meat. They are deficient in but one of the five food principles — namely, carbohydrates. From this fact, it may be plainly seen that they should be taken in combination with some starchy food, which furnishes the necessary bulk for the stomach.

The proteid found in the white of egg is nearly pure albumen. The yolk is of much greater nutritive value than the white. Its chemical composition is so complex that as yet it is but incompletely understood. It contains lime, calcium, iron, and phosphorus in organic combinations, which renders it readily absorbed and utilized by the body.

Eggs are expensive, even when obtained at twenty-five cents per dozen, but being so valuable a form of food,

# EGGS.

they should be used as freely as possible. They enter into the composition of many dishes to which they are indispensable.

Eggs for the sick should be as fresh as possible. If received from the market, packed in sawdust, they should be removed at once, as they quickly absorb odor from the wood, which gives to them an unpleasant flavor. If a patient should by chance be served an egg-nog made from a poor egg it might be difficult to persuade him to try another.

There are but few people with whom eggs disagree. If they cannot be taken it is usually due to the presence of lecithin, a nitrogenous, fatty substance found in the yolk which readily decomposes and forms acids. Convalescents, anæmics, and consumptives can take from six to eight eggs daily, for an extended period, with most satisfactory results, as they yield a large amount of nutriment for their bulk. For forced feeding they are most valuable, as they can be easily administered and combined with milk or broth.

Eggs deteriorate quickly in value unless air is excluded, which prevents the evaporation of water through the shell. By the evaporation of water air rushes in, causing decomposition. Various gases are given off, — principally, sulphuretted hydrogen, which may cause gastric and intestinal disorders.

### How preserved.

1. By the exclusion of air by coating, covering, or immersing.
2. By use of low temperature; that is, cold storage.

### Ways of determining Freshness of Eggs.

1. The shell of a freshly laid egg is slightly rough.
2. Shake egg in hand while holding to ear, and there should be but little sound.
3. Put in basin of water and they should sink.

Dealers determine the freshness of eggs by holding them in front of an electric light or lighted candle in a dark room. If they look clear the eggs are fresh; if a dark spot is in evidence the eggs are doubtful. The air space at the larger end of a freshly laid egg is quite small, but increases as the egg loses value. An egg deteriorates after twenty-four hours.

### Advantages of use in Sick-Room Cookery.

1. Nutritive value.
2. Taste good (if fresh).
3. Easily digested (if properly cooked).
4. Free from bacteria.
5. Contain practically no extractives.
6. Deficient in uric acid derivatives.
7. Hold lime, calcium, iron, and phosphorus in organic combination.
   Minerals in organic combination are more easily absorbed.
8. Fat in form of emulsion.

### Effects of Cooking.

The white of an egg being nearly pure albumen, serves as an excellent illustration for demonstrating the effect of heat on the principal constituent of proteid food. Illustrate by experiments.

1. Albumen is soluble in cold water.
2. Albumen is coagulated by hot water (134 to 167° F.) or by heat.
3. Albumen is coagulated by mineral acids.
4. Albumen is dissolved by vegetable acids.
   Exception, Cream of Tartar.
5. Albumen is coagulated by alcohol.

Albumen when acted upon by heat coagulates at a temperature of from 134 to 167° F.; herein lies the necessity of cooking eggs alone or in combination at a low temperature.

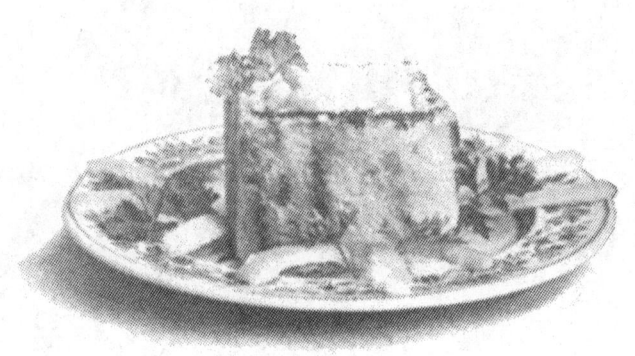

CROUSTADE OF CREAMED PEAS
See p. 157

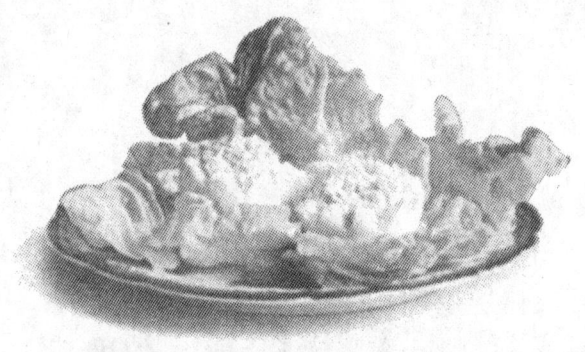

EGG SALAD
See p. 166

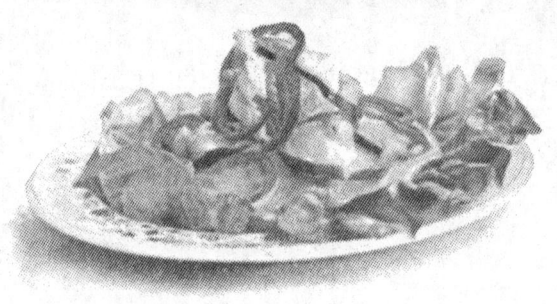

SWEETBREAD AND CELERY SALAD, GARNISHED WITH
RED AND GREEN PEPPER CUT IN NARROW STRIPS
See p. 168

The importance of this truth is best illustrated by the proper preparation of so-called "boiled eggs." If the egg is kept at a low temperature throughout the cooking, the white is soft and jelly like. Whereas, if the temperature is greatly increased, the white is tough and leathery. The yolk of the egg will cook at a relatively lower temperature than the white. In the former case the egg is readily digested; in the latter case it is difficult of digestion. Eggs for the sick, if served boiled, should be either soft or hard cooked, never midway between. If "hard boiled," the yolk may be reduced readily to a powder, which is not difficult of digestion.

### Digestibility.

Eggs are easily digested and well absorbed. Ninety-seven per cent of the proteid is absorbed and ninety-four per cent of the fat. A raw egg, on account of its blandness, does not stimulate the flow of gastric juice, consequently does not leave the stomach in so short a time as a "soft cooked" egg.

Two "soft boiled" eggs leave the stomach in one and three-fourths hours.

Two raw eggs leave the stomach in two and one-fourth hours.

Two "hard boiled" eggs (as commonly taken) leave the stomach in three hours. A "hard boiled" egg cooked at a low temperature (175° F.) for forty-five minutes, and chopped very finely, will leave the stomach almost as quickly as a "soft boiled" egg.

The digestibility of the white of an egg is increased by beating. By beating, the walls of the cells, which consist of albuminin, are ruptured, thus setting free the albumen, which is more quickly acted upon by the gastric juice.

## WAYS OF COOKING EGGS.

### "Soft Boiled" Egg I. 106 Calories.

Break egg into a china cup. Place cup in saucepan of hot water (175° F.), and as soon as white begins to cook, stir from sides of cup. using a silver spoon. When white is of jelly-like consistency, break yolk and mix with white. Add one teaspoon butter and a few grains salt. Serve in same cup.

### "Soft Boiled" Egg II.

Put an egg into a saucepan of hot water, using a spoon, allowing water to cover egg, and keeping water at a uniform temperature of 175° F. for six and one-half to eight minutes; or put egg in a saucepan of cold water, allowing water to heat gradually until boiling point is reached, time required for cooking being about the same. Remove egg from shell into a warm cup and add one teaspoon butter, and a few grains salt.

### "Hard Boiled" Egg.

Cook same as " Soft Boiled " Egg II. allowing egg to remain in water forty-five minutes. Finely chop, and add one teaspoon butter and a few grains salt.

### Dropped Egg I.

Butter inside of muffin ring and put in iron frying-pan of hot water to which one-half tablespoon salt has been added. Break egg into saucer, then slip into ring, allowing water to cover egg. Place on frying-pan a tin cover and set on back of range. Let stand until white of egg is of jelly-like consistency. Take up ring and egg, using a buttered griddle-cake turner, on to a circular piece of buttered toast. Remove ring and garnish egg with four toast points and parsley.

### Dropped Egg II.

Break egg into a large buttered mixing-spoon, immerse in a saucepan of hot water, and keep under water until white is of jelly-like consistency. Serve same as Dropped Egg I.

### Dropped Eggs with White Sauce. 265 Calories.

Heat a small omelet pan, place on asbestos mat, and set on back of range. Butter bottom and sides of pan, using one teaspoon butter, and turn in three-fourths cup scalded milk. Break egg into saucer, slip into pan, cover, cook on one side; turn, cover, and cook on other side. Remove egg to hot plate and thicken milk with one-half tablespoon each butter and flour worked together until thoroughly blended. Season with salt, and strain sauce around egg.

### Shirred Egg.

⅛ cup soft bread crumbs.  
½ tablespoon melted butter.  
1 egg.  
Few grains salt.

Mix bread crumbs and butter, stirring lightly with fork. Cover bottom of buttered egg-shirrer with crumbs, break egg, slip on to crumbs, sprinkle with salt, cover with crumbs, and bake in a moderate oven until white is set.

### Baked Egg. 220 Calories.

⅛ cup soft bread crumbs.  
1 tablespoon heavy cream.  
1 egg.  
Few grains salt.

Cover bottom of buttered egg-shirrer with crumbs. Break egg, slip on to crumbs, sprinkle with salt, pour over cream, cover with remaining crumbs, and bake same as Shirred Eggs.

### Scrambled Egg I. 137 Calories.

1 egg.  
½ tablespoon butter.  
1 tablespoon milk.  
Few grains salt.

Break egg, beat slightly, and add milk and salt. Heat omelet pan, put in butter, and when melted add mixture.

Cook until of creamy consistency, stirring and scraping from bottom and sides of pan.

### Scrambled Egg II.

1 egg.   ½ tablespoon butter.
Few grains salt.

Heat omelet pan, put in butter, and when melted, break egg into saucer, then slip into pan. Let stand until white is partially set, then break yolk, mix with white, and stir to finish the cooking. Sprinkle with salt.

### Coddled Egg.

1 egg.   1 teaspoon butter.
⅓ cup milk.   Salt.
Few grains pepper.

Scald milk, and add egg slightly beaten. Cook over hot water, stirring constantly until of a soft, creamy consistency, then add seasonings. Serve with toast points.

### Souffléd Egg.

Break egg and separate yolk from white. To white add few grains salt and beat until stiff, using Dover Egg Beater. Turn into a buttered glass and place on trivet in pan of hot water. Allow water to heat gradually until boiling point is reached, when egg should be cooked. As white of egg rises in cup, make a depression in centre and drop in yolk.

### Egg in a Nest.

Break egg and separate yolk from white. Beat white until stiff, using silver fork, then add a few grains salt. Pile on a circular piece of toasted bread, first dipped in boiling salted water; make depression in centre, and drop in yolk. Bake in a moderate oven until delicately browned. Serve with Béchamel Sauce, p. 150, or Tomato Sauce, p. 150.

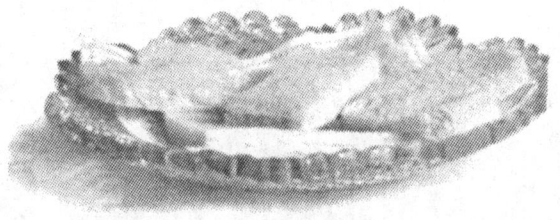

**BREAD AND BUTTER SANDWICHES**
See p. 169

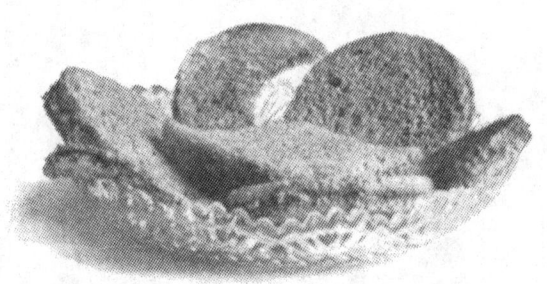

**ENTIRE WHEAT BREAD SANDWICHES**
See p. 169

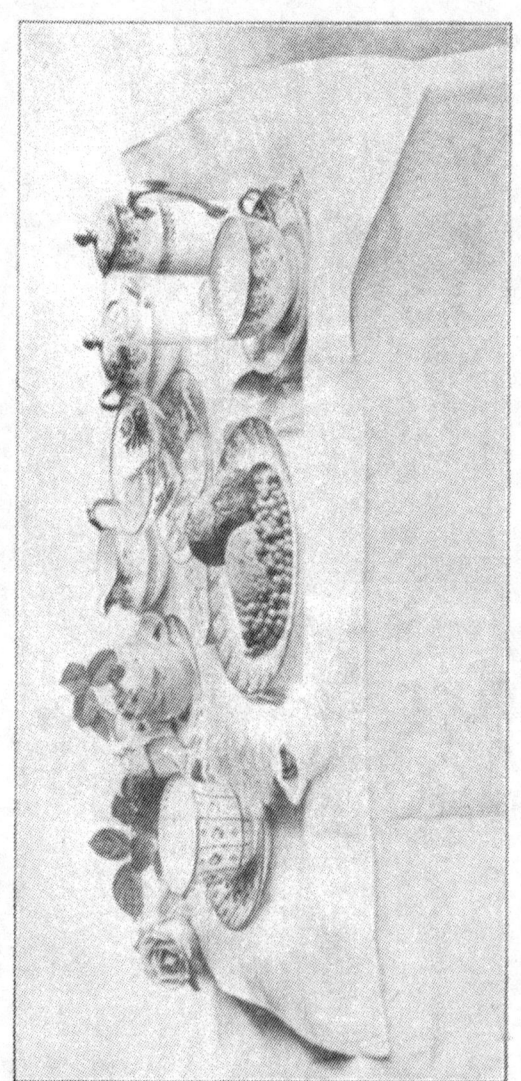

DINNER TRAY FOR THE CONVALESCENT

### Eggs à la Buckingham.

Serve Scrambled Egg I. or II. on one slice Cream Toast or Thickened Milk Toast.

### Egg Timbale.

| | |
|---|---|
| 1 teaspoon butter. | Yolk 1 egg. |
| 1 teaspoon flour. | White 1 egg. |
| ¼ cup scalded milk. | ⅛ teaspoon salt. |

Few grains celery salt.

Make sauce of butter, flour, and milk; cool, add yolk of egg, and beat two minutes. Beat white of egg until stiff and dry, and cut and fold into first mixture; turn into buttered mould, set in pan of hot water, and bake in slow oven until firm.

### Eggs à la Goldenrod.

| | |
|---|---|
| ½ cup scalded milk. | 1 hard boiled egg. |
| ½ tablespoon butter. | 2 slices bread. |
| ¾ tablespoon flour. | 6 toast points. |
| ¼ teaspoon salt. | Parsley. |

Make sauce of first four ingredients. Finely chop white of egg and reheat in sauce. Remove crust from bread, cut each slice in two, lengthwise, and toast until delicately browned. Arrange on serving-dish, pour over sauce. Cover sauce with yolk of egg forced through a strainer, and garnish with toast points and parsley.

### Egg Soufflé.

| | |
|---|---|
| ½ tablespoon butter. | Yolk 1 egg. |
| ½ tablespoon flour. | White 1 egg. |
| ⅓ cup scalded thin cream. | ¼ teaspoon salt. |

Work butter and flour together until well blended, pour on gradually the scalded cream. Cook in double boiler three minutes, cool slightly, add yolk of egg and salt, and beat two minutes, then cut and fold in white of egg beaten until stiff and dry. Turn into a buttered dish, set in pan of hot water, and bake in a slow oven until firm.

### Foamy Omelet I.

Yolk 1 egg. White 1 egg.
1 tablespoon cold water. ⅛ teaspoon salt.
½ teaspoon butter.

Add water to yolk of egg and beat until thick and lemon colored, using cup and smallest-sized egg-beater; then add salt and fold in white of egg beaten until stiff and dry. Heat omelet pan; butter bottom and sides of pan, turn in mixture, spread evenly with back of spoon, and cook slowly until delicately browned underneath. Place on centre grate in oven to finish cooking, which may be determined by pressure of finger; if omelet sticks to finger like beaten white of egg it is underdone; if it is firm to the touch it is ready to fold. Fold, turn on hot platter, and serve with or without white sauce.

Small omelet pans may be purchased of correct size for the cooking of one egg. The success of an omelet of this kind depends upon the amount of air inclosed in the egg and the expansion of that air in cooking.

### Foamy Omelet II.

Yolk 1 egg. White 1 egg.
¾ tablespoon hot water or milk. ⅛ teaspoon salt.
½ teaspoon butter.

Beat yolk of egg until thick and lemon colored, add water and salt. Do not stir mixture, but pour on to white of the egg beaten until stiff and dry; then cut and fold until white has taken up yolk and water. Cook same as Foamy Omelet I.

### Beef Omelet I.

Yolk 1 egg. White 1 egg.
¾ tablespoon boiling water. ⅛ teaspoon salt.
¼ teaspoon Liebig's Beef Extract. ½ teaspoon butter.

Dissolve beef extract in boiling water, and make same as Foamy Omelet II.

## Oyster Omelet.

| | |
|---|---|
| 1 cup oysters. | ¾ tablespoon flour. |
| 2 tablespoons cold water. | Scalded milk. |
| ¾ tablespoon butter. | Salt. |

Few grains pepper.

Make Foamy Omelet I. or II. Wash oysters by putting in strainer placed over bowl, pouring over water and picking over oysters carefully with the fingers. Reserve liquor, heat to boiling point, and strain through double thickness of cheese cloth. Melt butter, add flour, and pour on oyster liquor with enough milk to make one-half cup liquid. Parboil oysters until plump, drain, add oysters to sauce, and pour around omelet.

## Omelet with Peas.

| | |
|---|---|
| ¼ cup canned peas. | ¼ teaspoon sugar. |
| ½ tablespoon butter. | ¼ cup milk. |
| 1 teaspoon flour. | Few grains salt. |

Make Foamy Omelet I. or II. Rinse peas and put in small saucepan with butter; when thoroughly heated add flour and sugar, then add milk and salt. Be careful not to mash the peas by too much stirring. Serve around omelet. Asparagus tips or cauliflower may be used in place of peas.

## Bread Omelet.

| | |
|---|---|
| Yolk 1 egg. | White 1 egg. |
| 2 tablespoons stale bread crumbs. | ¼ teaspoon salt. |
| 2 tablespoons milk. | ¾ teaspoon butter. |

Add bread crumbs to milk and let stand until crumbs have taken up milk, then proceed same as in making Foamy Omelet II. adding bread to egg yolk.

### Beef Omelet II.

Yolk 1 egg.  
2 tablespoons stale bread crumbs.  
2 tablespoons boiling water.  
½ teaspoon Liebig's Beef Extract,  
   or 2 tablespoons strong beef stock.

White 1 egg.  
¼ teaspoon salt.  
¾ teaspoon butter  
Few grains celery salt.

Dissolve beef extract in boiling water, then proceed as in making Bread Omelet. Serve with or without Tomato Sauce.

### Cereal Omelet.

Yolk 1 egg.  
3 tablespoons warm mush of  
   Wheat, Rolled Oats, or Hominy.

White 1 egg.  
⅛ teaspoon salt.  
¾ teaspoon butter.

Follow directions for making Foamy Omelet II. Garnish with thin slices of cooked bacon.

### Jelly Omelet.

Follow directions for making Foamy Omelet I., adding one tablespoon powdered sugar and using only a few grains salt. When ready to fold spread one-half the upper surface with two tablespoons jelly (currant, grape, or crabapple) beaten with a fork. Fold, sprinkle top with powdered sugar, and score with a hot poker.

### Orange Omelet.

Yolk 1 egg.  
1 tablespoon orange juice.  
   Few grains salt.

White 1 egg.  
1 tablespoon powdered sugar.

Follow directions for making Foamy Omelet I. Serve garnished with sections of orange sprinkled with powdered sugar.

### French Omelet.

1 large egg.  
¾ tablespoon milk.

Few grains salt.  
½ tablespoon butter.

Beat egg with silver fork until yolk and white are blended, then add salt and milk. Heat omelet pan, add butter, and as soon as butter is melted, turn in mixture. As soon as it begins to cook, prick and pick up with fork, until it is of a creamy consistency throughout. Place on hotter part of range to brown underneath. Fold, and turn on hot plate. Garnish with parsley.

### Toast Meringue.

| | |
|---|---|
| 1 slice dry toast. | ½ teaspoon butter. |
| ½ cup cream. | Few grains salt. |

White 1 egg.

Heat cream in sauce pan placed on front of range. When cream is nearly at the boiling point add butter and the egg beaten until stiff, sprinkled with salt. Fold the egg over and over in the cream until firm, then pour all over the toast.

## CHAPTER XVII.

### SOUPS, BROTHS, AND STEWS.

SOUPS are usually divided into two great classes: —

1. Those made with stock.
2. Those made without stock.

Soups made with stock have for their basis beef, mutton, veal, poultry, fish or game, separately or in combination. They include bouillon, brown soup stock, consommé, lamb stock, and white soup stock. These should be made in large quantities and require much time and care in their preparation. Recipes may be found for the same in any reliable cook book.

Stock soups are valuable chiefly for their extractives. When taken as the first course of a dinner they stimulate gastric juice to such an extent that the solid foods which follow are much more readily digested than they otherwise would be. They are also useful to give variety to a liquid diet.

Soups without stock usually have as their basis cooked vegetables, forced through a strainer, diluted with stock and milk or milk alone. Cream soups have a food value, largely due to the milk and butter which they contain, the vegetables being added for the purpose of giving flavor, with the exception of peas and beans, which increase nutritive value.

#### Potato Soup I. 232 Calories.

$2/3$ cup milk.
$1/6$ slice onion.
$1/4$ cup hot mashed potato.
$1/2$ tablespoon butter.
$1/2$ tablespoon flour.
$1/4$ teaspoon salt.
Few grains pepper.
Few grains celery salt.

Scald milk with onion, remove onion, and add milk slowly to potatoes. Melt butter, add flour and seasonings,

# SOUPS, BROTHS, AND STEWS.

stir until well mixed, then pour on gradually hot mixture. Bring to boiling point, strain, and serve. Soup may be sprinkled with finely chopped parsley if desired.

### Potato Soup II.

Follow directions for Potato Soup I. and add just before serving one teaspoon tomato catsup.

### Cream of Pea Soup.

⅓ cup canned peas.
¼ cup cold water.
¼ teaspoon sugar.
⅔ cup scalded milk.
¼ tablespoon butter.
¾ tablespoon flour.
⅛ teaspoon salt.
Few grains pepper.

Drain peas from their liquor, rinse thoroughly, add sugar and cold water, and simmer ten minutes. Rub through a sieve, and thicken with butter and flour cooked together; add milk and seasonings. Strain into a hot cup, and serve with Croûtons.

### Mock Bisque. 153 Calories.

⅔ cup milk.
¾ tablespoon flour.
Cold water.
¼ teaspoon sugar.
¼ cup stewed and steamed tomatoes.
Few grains soda.
Few grains pepper.
½ tablespoon butter.
¼ teaspoon salt.

Scald milk and thicken with flour diluted with cold water until thin enough to pour. Cook over hot water ten minutes, stirring constantly at first. Heat tomatoes to boiling point, add soda and sugar, and then add gradually to thickened milk. Add butter in small pieces and salt; then strain. If not served at once soup is liable to curdle.

### Asparagus Soup. 86 Calories.

10 stalks of asparagus, or
⅓ cup asparagus tips.
⅔ cup chicken stock.
Yolk 1 egg.
1 tablespoon heavy cream.
⅛ teaspoon salt.
Few grains pepper.

Drain asparagus tips from their liquor, cover with cold water, and bring to boiling point, then drain. Add asparagus to stock, and let simmer ten minutes; rub through a sieve, reheat, add egg yolk, cream, and seasoning. Strain before serving.

### Cream of Corn Soup.

⅓ cup canned corn.
⅓ cup boiling water.
⅔ cup milk.
¼ slice onion.
½ tablespoon butter.
¾ tablespoon flour.
¼ teaspoon salt.
Few grains pepper.

Chop corn, add water, and simmer ten minutes; rub through a sieve. Scald milk with onion, remove onion, and thicken milk with butter and flour cooked together. Add seasonings, and strain

### Cream of Celery Soup. 276 Calories.

1 stalk celery.
⅔ cup milk.
½ tablespoon butter.
¾ tablespoon flour.
¼ cup cream.
Salt and pepper.

Break celery in pieces and pound in a mortar. Add to milk, and cook in double boiler twenty minutes. Thicken with butter and flour cooked together, season, add cream, strain, and serve.

### Spinach Soup.

1 tablespoon chopped cooked spinach.
⅓ cup white stock.
⅓ cup milk.
½ tablespoon butter.
¾ tablespoon flour.
Salt.
Pepper.

Add spinach to stock, heat to boiling point, and rub through a sieve. Thicken with butter and flour cooked together, add milk and seasonings, reheat, strain, and serve. The water in which a fowl or chicken is cooked makes white stock.

### Cauliflower Soup.

¼ cup cooked cauliflower.
⅓ cup white stock.
⅓ cup milk.
½ tablespoon butter.
¾ tablespoon flour.
Salt.
Pepper.

Make same as Spinach Soup.

# SOUPS, BROTHS, AND STEWS.

### Tomato Soup. 100 Calories.

⅔ cup tomatoes
   (canned or fresh).
⅓ cup water.
3 peppercorns.
1 clove

¼ teaspoon sugar.
⅙ slice onion.
¼ teaspoon salt.
Few grains soda.
½ tablespoon butter.

¾ tablespoon flour.

Mix first six ingredients and cook ten minutes. Rub through sieve, add salt and soda, thicken with butter and flour cooked together, and strain.

### Oyster Stew. 219 Calories.

⅔ cup scalded milk.
½ cup oysters.
1 tablespoon water.

⅓ teaspoon salt.
Few grains pepper.
½ tablespoon butter.

Put oysters in strainer placed over bowl, pour over water; and carefully pick over oysters, removing all particles of shell. Pour liquor from bowl to saucepan, and heat to boiling point; strain through double cheese cloth, return to saucepan, add oysters, and cook until oysters are plump and edges curl. Remove oysters to warm bowl, add butter, salt, and pepper, oyster liquor strained a second time, and milk. Serve with small finger-shaped pieces of toast piled log-cabin fashion.

### Oyster Soup.

½ cup oysters.
½ cup milk
Small stalk celery.
Bit of parsley.
Bit of bay leaf.

⅙ slice onion.
½ tablespoon butter.
¾ tablespoon flour.
¼ teaspoon salt.
Few grains pepper.

Finely chop oysters, put in saucepan, and heat slowly to boiling point. Strain through double thickness cheese cloth, reserve liquor, and thicken with butter and flour cooked together. Scald milk with celery, parsley, bay leaf, and onion; then strain. Add to first mixture, season, and strain. Serve with croûtons.

### Clam Soup.

| | |
|---|---|
| 1 doz. soft-shelled clams. | ¾ tablespoon flour. |
| ½ cup scalded milk. | ⅛ teaspoon salt. |
| ¾ tablespoon butter. | Few grains pepper. |

Wash and scrub clams, changing the water several times. Put in saucepan with two tablespoons water and cook until shells open. Remove clams from shells, reserve soft portions and liquor drained from clams. Strain liquor through double thickness cheese cloth, reheat, and thicken with butter and flour cooked together. Add milk, soft part of clams, salt, and pepper.

### Triplex Soup.

Use equal quantities of beef, lamb, or mutton and veal, allowing one pint water to each pound of meat. Cut meat in small pieces, add cold water, heat slowly to boiling point, skim, and let simmer four hours. Strain, cool, remove fat, and reheat for serving. Season with salt.

Doctors frequently order this soup for patients.

### Mutton Broth.

| | |
|---|---|
| 3 lbs. lamb, cut from forequarter. | 2 tablespoons boiled rice, or barley. |
| 3 pints cold water. | 1 teaspoon salt. |

Wipe meat, remove from bones, discard skin and fat, and cut lean meat in small pieces. Put meat and bones in kettle, add water, heat gradually to boiling point, skim, and cook slowly until meat is tender. Add salt when half cooked. Strain, remove fat, reheat, and add cooked rice. It is sometimes desirable to force rice through a purée strainer. It is more satisfactory to cook rice separately in boiling salted water before adding to broth. If cooked in broth it absorbs a large quantity of the liquid. When barley is used, soak over night or several hours before cooking. A few mint leaves or a sprig of parsley may be added to give additional flavor.

### Chicken Broth.

3½ lb. chicken.   2 tablespoons rice.
3 pints cold water.   1½ teaspoons salt.
Few grains pepper.

Clean chicken; remove skin and fat, disjoint, and wipe with a wet cloth. Put in kettle, add cold water, heat slowly to boiling point, skim, and cook until meat is tender. Add salt and pepper when half cooked. Strain, and remove fat. Reheat to boiling point, add rice, and cook until rice is soft It is sometimes necessary to cook rice separately, and rub through a sieve before adding to broth.

### Chicken Broth with Cream.

Prepare same as Chicken Broth, and reduce stock to one quart. Omit rice, and allow one tablespoon heavy cream to a cup of stock. A few grains celery salt may be added to give additional flavor.

### Chicken Broth with Egg. 70 Calories.

Beat one egg slightly, and pour on gradually while stirring constantly one cup hot chicken stock. Cook one minute and strain. Care must be taken that egg does not be over-cooked, as broth would have a curdled appearance.

### Chicken Purée.

⅓ cup chopped cooked fowl.   2 tablespoons butter.
1 cup scalded milk.   Salt.

Force meat through a purée strainer, then pound in a mortar. Add butter, and, gradually, scalded milk. Season to taste with salt.

## SOUP ACCOMPANIMENTS.

### Crisp Crackers.

Split common crackers and spread with butter, using one-fourth teaspoon butter to each one-half cracker. Place in pan and bake in a moderate oven until delicately browned.

### Croûtons.

Cut one slice bread one-third inch thick, remove crusts, butter sparingly, cut in strips one-third inch wide, and strips in cubes. Put in pan and bake in a moderate oven until delicately browned. To be served with Cream Soups.

### Imperial Sticks.

Cut stale bread in one-third inch slices, remove crusts, butter sparingly, and cut in one-third inch strips. Place in pan and bake in a moderate oven until delicately browned.

Cut stale bread in slices, shape with circular cutters, making rings. Spread rings sparingly with butter and brown in oven. Slip three imperial sticks through each ring.

## CHAPTER XVIII.

### FISH.

FISH, commonly speaking, is sea food. Fish is at its best when fresh, and in season. It should be eaten as soon as possible after being taken from the water. If fish is fresh the eyes and gills are bright, the tail firm, the flesh hard, and the scales do not come off easily.

Fish may be classified:

I. Scaly.
    1. White fish (fat secreted in liver).
        Examples: haddock, halibut, turbot, flounder, etc.
    2. Oily fish (fat deposited throughout the body).
        Examples: bluefish, eels, mackerel, salmon, etc.

II. Shell Fish.
    1. Mollusks. Examples: oysters, clams, etc.
    2. Crustaceans. Examples: crab, lobster, and shrimp.

The proteid and fat of fish, as of meat, are their chief nutritive constituents. A large amount of the proteid of fish is in the form of gelatin. Fish is less rich in extractives and less stimulating than meat, for which reason people tire of it more quickly. It offers variety rather than furnishes a constant diet. Fish is less nutritious than meat, with the exception of the oily fish, — salmon, eels, herrings, etc.

The popular fallacy that fish is a brain food is unfounded. As a matter of fact many kinds of meat contain more phosphorus than any kind of fish. There is **no special brain food.**

### Table showing Composition of Fish allowed for the Convalescent.

| Article. | Refuse. | Proteid. | Fat. | Mineral matter. | Water. |
|---|---|---|---|---|---|
| Cod, salt, boneless | | 22.2 | .3 | 23.1 | 54.4 |
| Flounder | 61.5 | 5.6 | .3 | .5 | 32.1 |
| Haddock | 51. | 8.2 | .2 | .6 | 40. |
| Halibut | 17.7 | 15.1 | 4.4 | .9 | 61.9 |
| Mackerel, Spanish | 34.6 | 13.7 | 6.2 | 1. | 44.5 |
| Perch, white | 62.5 | 7.2 | 1.5 | .4 | 28.4 |
| Salmon | 39.2 | 12.4 | 8.1 | .9 | 39.4 |
| Shad | 50.1 | 9.2 | 4 8 | .7 | 35.2 |
| Smelts | 41.9 | 10. | 1. | 1. | 46.1 |
| Trout | 48.1 | 9.8 | 1.1 | .6 | 40.4 |
| Turbot | 47.7 | 6.8 | 7.5 | .7 | 37.3 |
| Whitefish | 53.5 | 10.3 | 3. | .7 | 32.5 |

| Article. | Refuse. | Proteid. | Fat. | Mineral matter. | Carbohydrates. | Water. |
|---|---|---|---|---|---|---|
| Lobsters | 61.7 | 5.9 | .7 | .8 | .2 | 30.7 |
| Clams, out of shell | | 10.6 | 1.1 | 2.3 | 5.2 | 80.8 |
| Oysters, solid | | 6.1 | 1.4 | .9 | 3.3 | 88 3 |

Prof W. O. Atwater.

Under scaly fish, white fish is the only class usually considered in invalid cookery. Exception must be made to codfish, which on account of its coarse fibre is never allowed. During advanced convalescence, oily fish may be occasionally introduced into the dietary.

Oysters, among mollusks, take first rank. The five food principles are represented in their composition, and in about the same proportion as in milk.

Their carbohydrate is in the form of glycogen (animal starch). Milk has the advantage over oysters as a food, as it is much cheaper and may be taken in large quantities. Oysters are taken in such limited numbers they furnish a comparatively small amount of nutriment; they are, however, if eaten raw, very easily digested. They offer a pleasing variety to the diet on account of their delicious flavor. They may be cooked

# FISH.

in a great variety of ways, which enables them to be used to advantage.

Frequently oysters are of a greenish color, which is due not to parasites, as many suppose, but to the green coloring matter in the plant on which the oysters have fed.

Oysters are in season from September to May. During the remaining months, which is their breeding season, they are flabby and of inferior flavor. While many believe them to be injurious when out of season, this is not the case, if they are eaten soon after being taken from the oyster beds.

Clams are similar in composition to oysters, but are not so generally used, nor so well liked. They contain a tough portion, which should be discarded in sick-room cookery.

While analysis shows the nutritive value of lobsters to be considerable, they are coarse feeders, which renders the fibre dense and close, making them difficult of digestion. Lobsters, on account of their price, must be considered as a delicacy, except in places where they are abundant, and even in such places lobsters of short length are frequently sold, which is contrary to law. The United States is endeavoring to protect the lobster industry by forbidding the sale of all lobsters under certain lengths, (which lengths differ in different states), ten inches being the shortest.

As a rule, the use of lobsters in the sick-room should not be considered. To many they are poisonous, and to others with whom they agree they have a decidedly appetizing effect; to the latter class they are allowed occasionally during convalescence.

Salt codfish, on account of its low price and high nutritive value, is a most important form of food. When finely divided and served as creamed codfish, it may furnish the principal dish to a most satisfactory meal.

## Cooking of.

The same principles which apply to the cooking of meat apply also to the cooking of fish, and the same methods

FOOD AND COOKERY.

for cooking should be employed. Fish, being less rich in extractives than meat, usually needs the accompaniment of some kind of a sauce.

### Digestibility.

White fish, as a rule, are more easily digested than beef, lamb, or chicken. For this reason their use is often recommended for those of sedentary habits. They furnish a desirable substitute for the more stimulating meats during warm weather.

Oily fish are digested with about the same ease and in about the same time as meats containing a relatively small quantity of fat.

Salt fish is less easily digested than other fish, due to the fact that the fibre is hardened during the process of salting.

While there is a tendency to carry personal idiosyncrasies too far, there are undoubtedly many by whom fish cannot be taken. It acts as a poison, oftentimes producing diseases of the skin. There are others with whom the fat of fish disagrees, causing acidity and eructation of the stomach.

## WAYS OF COOKING.

### Steamed Halibut.

Clean a small piece of halibut by wiping with a cheese cloth wrung out of cold water. Put in strainer, and place over a kettle of boiling water, cover closely, and keep water at boiling point until fish is done. The fish is cooked when flesh leaves the bone. Remove to hot serving-dish, take off outside skin, and pour around

DRAWN BUTTER SAUCE. Melt three-fourths tablespoon butter, add three-fourths tablespoon flour, and when well mixed pour on gradually, while stirring constantly, one-half cup boiling water. Season with salt, then add three-fourths tablespoon butter in small pieces, and one-half " hard boiled " egg cut in thin slices.

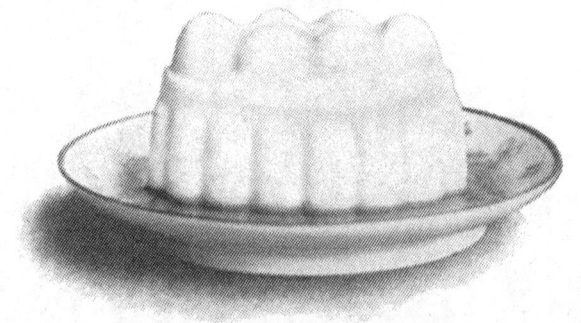

RICE JELLY WITH FRUIT SAUCE
See p. 179

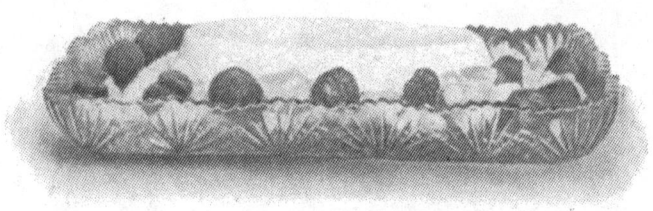

FRUIT BLANC MANGE
See p. 186

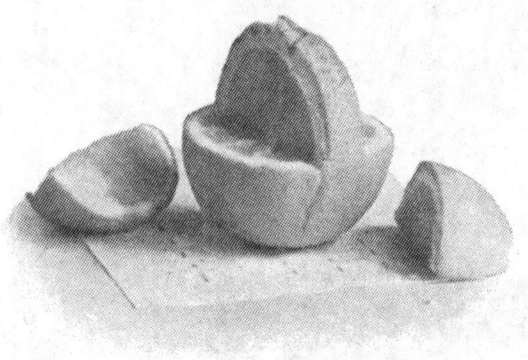

**FIRST STEP IN MAKING ORANGE BASKET**
See p. 181

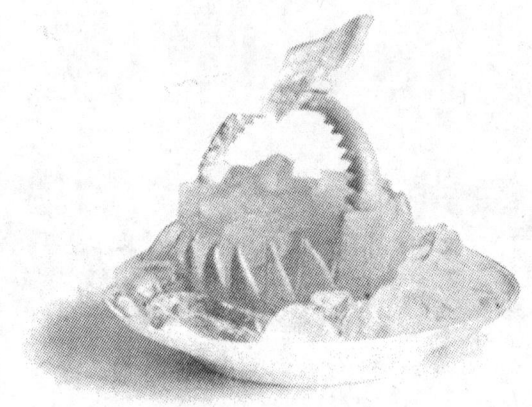

**ORANGE BASKET**
See p. 181

### Boiled Haddock.

Clean and wipe a small piece of haddock, then tie in cheese cloth. Put on trivet placed in stewpan of boiling water to which has been added one tablespoon each salt and vinegar, having water cover fish.

Salt adds to the flavor; vinegar helps to keep the fish white. Cook until flesh separates from bone, the time required being about fifteen minutes. Place on hot serving-dish, remove skin, garnish with parsley, and serve with

EGG SAUCE. Melt three-fourths tablespoon butter, add three-fourths tablespoon flour, and pour on gradually one-half cup scalded milk. Beat yolk one egg, dilute with one tablespoon hot mixture, add to remaining mixture, and season with salt.

### Broiled Fish.

Smelts and other small fish are broiled whole, sometimes being split; while larger fish are cut in slices three-fourths inch in thickness for broiling.

Wipe fish, sprinkle with salt, and put in buttered wire broiler, place over hot fire, turning every ten seconds during the first minute of the cooking (to coagulate the albuminous juices, thus preventing their escape), and afterwards occasionally.

When fish is thoroughly heated, brush over, without unlocking broiler, with melted butter, first on one side then on the other. Cook until well browned on both sides, remove to hot serving-dish, sprinkle with salt, spread with soft butter, and garnish with parsley and lemon cut in fancy shapes.

Small fish, when spilt for broiling, should be first broiled on flesh side, then turned and browned on skin side just long enough to make skin brown and crisp. To remove fish from broiler, loosen fish on one side, turn, and loosen on other side, using a three-tined fork.

130    FOOD AND COOKERY.

### Baked Fillets of Halibut.

Remove skin and bones from one-half slice of halibut, leaving two fillets. Fasten in shape with small wooden skewers, sprinkle with salt, brush over with lemon juice, cover, and let stand twenty minutes. Put in pan, brush over with melted butter, cover with buttered paper, and bake twelve minutes in a hot oven. Remove to hot serving-dish, garnish with yolk of "hard boiled" egg, forced through a strainer, and white of egg cut in rings, strips, or fancy shapes. Serve with Egg Sauce, to which is added a few drops lemon juice.

### Creamed Fish.

$\frac{1}{4}$ cup cold cooked flaked fish.  $\frac{1}{4}$ cup milk.
1 teaspoon butter.    3 drops onion juice.
1 teaspoon flour.    Salt.

Make sauce of butter, flour, and milk; season with onion juice and salt, add fish, and reheat.

Creamed Fish may be served attractively in a potato border.

### Scalloped Fish.

Put Creamed Fish in buttered individual baking-dish, cover with buttered crumbs, and bake until crumbs are brown. For buttered crumbs allow one-half cracker and one-half teaspoon melted butter.

### Halibut Timbale.

Wipe small piece uncooked halibut, remove skin and bones, and force fish through a purée strainer; there should be one-fourth cup. Add one-fourth teaspoon flour, one-third egg yolk, and two tablespoons heavy cream. Season with salt and paprika. Turn into individual moulds, set in pan of hot water, cover with buttered paper, and bake, in a moderate oven, until firm. Turn on hot serving-dish and pour around one-third cup White Sauce (see p. 148) to which is added two tablespoons peas, canned or freshly cooked.

## Fish Soufflé.

Force cooked fish through a purée strainer; there should be one-fourth cup. Cook one-fourth cup stale bread crumbs with one-third cup milk five minutes. Add fish, one-half tablespoon butter, and salt and paprika. Beat white of one small egg until stiff, add to mixture, and turn into two buttered individual moulds. Cook same as Halibut Timbale. Serve with White Sauce (see p. 148).

### Creamed Codfish.

¼ cup salt codfish.  ½ tablespoon flour.
½ tablespoon butter.  ⅓ cup scalded milk.
Yolk ½ egg.

Pick fish in pieces, cover with lukewarm water, and let stand until fish is soft. Drain from water, and add to sauce made of butter, flour, and milk. Just before serving add yolk of egg slightly beaten. Care must be taken that egg does not become overcooked. Should this happen, sauce will have a curdled appearance. Pour over a slice of toast, or serve with baked potato.

### Raw Oysters.

Serve six raw oysters on deep halves of the shells. Arrange on plate of crushed ice with one-fourth lemon in the centre of plate. Salt and pepper should accompany raw oysters.

### Raw Oysters with Sherry.

Put six raw oysters in glass, sprinkle with salt, and pour over one tablespoon sherry. An unsweetened wafer cracker should accompany this dish.

### Oysters baked in Shells.

Wash and scrub six oysters in shell. Arrange in a small tin on a bed of rock salt. Put in hot oven, and bake until shells begin to open. Remove shallow halves of shells, leaving oysters in deep halves. Arrange on serving-dish, sprinkle with salt and pepper, and season with butter.

The rock salt is used to balance the shells in such a position that the oyster liquor may not escape.

### Fancy Roast.

½ cup oysters.  Few grains pepper.
½ tablespoon butter.  3 slices toast.
Few grains salt.

Wash and pick over oysters. Drain, put in small omelet pan and cook over hot fire until oysters are plump and edges begin to curl, shaking pan occasionally, or stirring oysters with a silver fork. Add butter, salt, and pepper, reheat, and pour over one slice toast; cut remaining slices so as to leave two large toast points. Arrange toast points to meet over centre of oysters. Garnish with parsley.

How to wash Oysters. Put oysters in strainer, place strainer over bowl and pour over cold water, allowing one tablespoon to each half cup of oysters. Carefully pick over oysters, taking each one separately in the fingers, and remove any particle of shell which adheres to tough muscle.

### Grilled Oysters.

Wash and pick over one-half cup oysters, put in small omelet pan, and as fast as liquor flows, remove with a spoon; so continue until oysters are plump and edges begin to curl. Sprinkle oysters with salt and pepper, add one-half tablespoon butter, and pour over piece of toast or zephyrettes.

### Oyster Fricassee.

Wash and pick over one-half cup oysters, reserve liquor, heat gradually to boiling point, and strain through double thickness of cheese cloth. Add oysters to liquor

## FISH.

and cook until plump, then remove with a spoon. Add enough cream to oyster liquor to make one-third cup. Melt one-half tablespoon butter, add one-half tablespoon flour, and pour on gradually the liquor. Add oysters, season with salt and pepper, add yolk one-half egg slightly beaten, pour over toast, and sprinkle with one-fourth teaspoon finely chopped parsley.

### Creamed Oysters.

½ cup oysters.  
¾ tablespoon butter.  
1 tablespoon flour.  
⅓ cup scalded milk.  
Few grains salt.  
"    "  pepper.  
Few grains celery salt.

Wash, and pick over oysters, then cook until plump and edges curl. Drain, and add to sauce made of remaining ingredients. Sauce may be made of half oyster liquor and half milk or cream, if preferred. Serve on slices of toast or in Croustades of Bread (see p. 99).

### Broiled Oysters.

4 large selected oysters.  
¼ cup cracker crumbs.  
1½ tablespoons melted butter.  
Salt.  
Pepper.

Wash and pick over oysters, then drain and dry between towels. Put cup containing butter in saucepan of hot water. Take up each oyster separately by means of tough muscle, using a silver fork, dip in melted butter, then in seasoned cracker crumbs. Place on a buttered fine wire broiler and broil over a clear fire, turning often until slightly browned and the juices begin to flow. Arrange on serving-dish and garnish with parsley and a piece of lemon.

### Celeried Oysters.

Arrange Broiled Oysters on small pieces of Dipped Toast (see p. 99) and sprinkle with finely chopped celery.

## CHAPTER XIX.

### MEAT.

MEAT, commonly speaking, is flesh food. Examples: beef, mutton, veal, pork, poultry, game, etc., etc.

**Table showing Composition of Meats used for the Sick.**

| Articles. | Refuse. | Proteid. | Fat. | Mineral matter. | Water. |
|---|---|---|---|---|---|
| BEEF. | | | | | |
| Fore-quarter | 19.8 | 14.1 | 16.1 | .7 | 49.3 |
| Hind-quarter | 16.3 | 15.3 | 15.6 | .8 | 52. |
| Round | 8.5 | 18.7 | 8.8 | 1. | 63. |
| Rump | 18.5 | 14.4 | 19. | .8 | 47.3 |
| Loin | 12.6 | 15.9 | 17.3 | .9 | 53.3 |
| Chuck ribs | 13.3 | 15. | 20.8 | .8 | 50.1 |
| MUTTON. | | | | | |
| Hind-quarter | 16.7 | 13.5 | 23.5 | .7 | 45.6 |
| Fore-quarter | 21.1 | 11.9 | 25.7 | .7 | 40.6 |
| Leg | 17.4 | 15.1 | 14.5 | .8 | 52.2 |
| Loin | 14.2 | 12.8 | 31.9 | .6 | 40.5 |
| PORK. | | | | | |
| Ham, smoked | 12.7 | 14.1 | 33.2 | 4.1 | 35.9 |
| Salt pork | 8.1 | 6.5 | 66.8 | 2.7 | 15.9 |
| Bacon | 8.1 | 9.6 | 60.2 | 4.3 | 17.8 |
| POULTRY. | | | | | |
| Chicken | 34.8 | 14.8 | 1.1 | .8 | 48.5 |
| Fowl | 30. | 13.4 | 10.2 | .8 | 45.6 |
| Turkey | 22.7 | 15.7 | 18.4 | .8 | 42.4 |
| Sweetbread | | 15.4 | 12.1 | 1.6 | 70.9 |

PROF. W. O. ATWATER.

## MEAT.

### Structure of Meat.

Meat is made up of bundles of fibres (tube-shaped cells) containing water which holds in solution proteids, extractives, and salt to such an extent that the whole is jelly-like in consistency. The walls of the cells consist of an albuminoid substance called elastin. The bundles of fibres are held together by connective tissue, a gelatinous substance called collogen.

Between the fibres is a fluid which holds soluble albumen.

The proteid of meat consists of different nitrogenous substances which take different names: Myosin, the basis of muscle; fibrin, found in the muscle and the blood; and albumen, found in the blood and juices. Fibrin causes blood to clot. Gelatin is obtained from connective tissue, tendon, cartilage, and bone by boiling with water. Collogen is the name given to gelatin in its raw state. Gelatin, although highly nitrogenous, cannot fill the place of albumen, but spares it to such an extent that it is ranked in food classification among the proteids. It is capable of building tissues to a small extent, when taken in large quantities.

All meats contain extractives. They have a stimulating effect upon the system, and while they have but little food value, are of great importance, as to them is due the characteristic flavor of all meats. Pawlow writes: "They are the most powerful exciters of gastric secretion." The flesh of mature animals is richer in extractives than the flesh of young animals.

The fat of meat is intermingled with the lean portion or occurs in masses under the skin or about the internal organs. The nutritive value of meat depends largely upon the quantity of fat it contains. The larger the proportion of fat, the smaller the proportion of water, the fat supplementing the water.

Phosphoric acid and potash are the chief mineral substances found in meat. They are very valuable as build-

136 FOOD AND COOKERY.

ing material, and where there is an insufficient supply the muscles are poorly developed.

The proteid of meat is the most expensive form in which proteid can be obtained, unless it be from the cheapest cuts. Cheap cuts, if properly cooked, are as

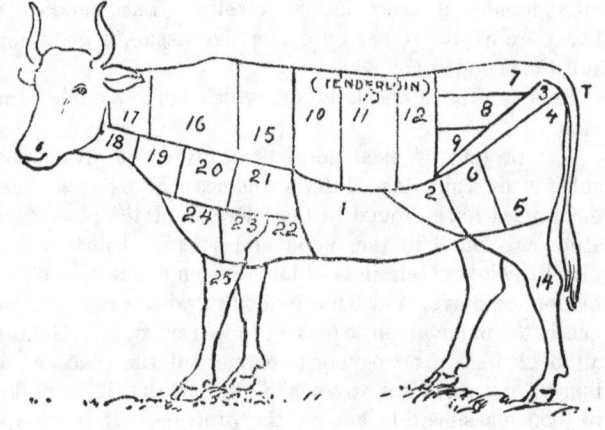

A SIDE OF BEEF.

easily digested and well absorbed as the more expensive ones, and their use should be encouraged. The art of good cookery is here well emphasized.

### Beef.

Beef ranks first among meats as regards nutritive value and consumption. This may be due in part to the fact that people tire less quickly of it than of other meats. The opinion is held that the red meats hold the more extractives, consequently are more stimulating than the white meats: this, however, is repudiated by Van Noorden, who claims there is little difference between red and white meats extractives.

## MEAT.

### A Side of Beef.

#### HIND-QUARTER.

Divisions.

1. Flank — Thick.
2. — Boneless.
3. — Aitch Bone.
4. Round — Top.
5. — Lower Part.
6. — Vein.
7. Rump — Back.
8. — Middle.
9. — Face.
10. Loin — Tip.
11. — Middle.
12. — First cut.
13. The Tenderloin — Sometimes sold as a fillet.
14. Hind-Shin

#### FORE-QUARTER.

15. Five Prime Ribs.
16. Five Chuck Ribs.
17. Neck.
18. Sticking-Piece.
19. Rattle Rand — Thick End.
20. — Second Cut.
21. — Thin End.
22. Brisket — Navel End.
23. — Butt End or
24. — Fancy Brisket.
25. Fore-Shin.

### How to determine Good Beef.

The quality of beef depends upon the breed, environment, age, and care in feeding of the animal, and also the manner of transportation and the time of hanging of the meat. The best beef is obtained from a steer of four or five years of age. The creature should hang after killing from two to three weeks. During this time lactic acid is formed, which acts upon the connective tissue, and the meat becomes tender and develops new flavors. First quality beef is firm and of fine-grained texture, bright red in color, and well mottled and coated with fat. The fat is firm and of a yellowish color.

Veal is obtained from the calf, and should never be used in the sick-room except for the making of broths. It comes from an immature animal, therefore contains but little nutritive value, and is difficult of digestion, in this latter respect being an exception to the general rule.

A sweetbread, the thymus gland of the calf, consists of two parts connected by tubing and membrane. The round compact part is called the heart sweetbread; the other portion, the throat sweetbread. They should never be bought disconnected, as the heart sweetbread is the more desirable. A sweetbread is made up of proteid and fat with but little connective tissue. Its proteid contains nuclein, which in digestion gives rise to uric acid derivatives; therefore its use should be restricted in the dietary of a patient who already has an excess of uric acid in the system.

Sweetbreads are the most easily digested of all meats, with but one exception, namely, calf's brains, which are very poorly absorbed. Sweetbreads are in season during the late spring and early summer. While they are obtainable throughout the year, they are very expensive in city markets when out of season.

### Mutton and Lamb.

Mutton is commonly ranked next to beef in nutritive value and consumption. According to some authorities it holds an equal place, and English writers on the subject often give it the preference. All agree that the fat of mutton is more difficult of digestion than the fat of beef. Lamb is young mutton. When coming from a creature killed at the age of from six weeks to three months, it is called spring lamb. Spring lamb appears in the market as early as February or March, and commands a very high price.

### How to determine Good Mutton and Lamb.

First-quality mutton comes from a sheep about three years old, and like beef should be allowed to hang to ripen and develop flavor. Good mutton is fine grained, bright pink in color, and the fat is hard, white, and flaky. If the skin comes off easily, mutton is sure to be good. Lamb should not be allowed to hang, but should be sold soon after killing. A leg of lamb may be distinguished from a leg of mutton, as the bone at the joint is serrated, rather than smooth and rounded. Lamp chops may be readily distinguished from mutton chops by the red color of the bone. As the creature grows old the blood recedes from the bone, therefore in mutton the bone is white. A lamb one year old is called a yearling, and furnishes lamb, while an older animal furnishes mutton.

### Pork.

Pork as ordinarily considered is the most difficult of digestion of all meats, and in health should seldom be used, while in the sick-room it should never be permitted. Many cases of ptomaine poisoning have been reported from its use. Exception must be made, however, to ham, salt pork, and bacon. A thin slice of broiled ham, baked bacon, or broiled salt pork are well borne by people in the early stages of convalescence, the salty taste acting as a stimulant to restore lost appetite. The manner of cutting and cooking is of the utmost importance.

### Poultry and Game.

Poultry includes the domestic birds, while game includes the birds and animals which are hunted for food.

Chicken, fowl, turkey, squab, and quail are allowed in the dietary of the sick.

A chicken is recognized by its soft feet, smooth skin, soft cartilage at the end of the breastbone, and frequently, by the abundance of pin-feathers.

In fowl the feet are hard and dry, the cartilage at the end of the breastbone is firm, and pin-feathers have given place to long hairs.

Chicken is more easily digested than fowl, but has not so great nutritive value. The breast of chicken has very short fibres, a small amount of connective tissue, and is practically free from fat. It is one of the most easily digested cuts of meat. Squabs and quails are likewise easily digested, and may be introduced into the dietary of a convalescent quite as early as chicken.

### Effects of Cooking.

Stewing, broiling, roasting, and baking are the methods employed in the cooking of meats for the sick.

The method depends on the cut as well as the result to be obtained.

In the cooking there is a loss of water, mineral matter, fat, and some extractives, the greatest loss being in water; consequently cooked meat represents more nutritive value, weight for weight, than raw meat.

### Losses in Cooking.

|  | Boiling. | Baking. | Broiling. |
|---|---|---|---|
| 4 lbs. of beef lose in weight | 1 lb. | 1 lb. 3 oz. | 1 lb. 5 oz. |
| 4 lbs. mutton lose in weight | 14 oz. | 1 lb. 4 oz. | 1 lb. 6 oz. |

JOHNSTON.

### Comparative Composition of Beef before and after Cooking.

|  | Water. | Nitrogenous matter. | Fat. | Extractives. | Salts. |
|---|---|---|---|---|---|
| Raw | 70.88% | 22.51% | 4.52% | .86% | 1.23% |
| Same after boiling | 56.82% | 34.13% | 7.50% | .40% | 1.15% |
| Same after broiling | 55.39% | 34.23% | 8.21% | .72% | 1.45% |

KÖNIG.

Cold water draws out the soluble albumen, the extractives, and some of the salts of meat. By gradually raising the temperature and keeping it at 185° F. for several hours, gelatin is obtained from connective tissue and

MEAT. 141

bone. In soup making this is the object to be accomplished. When meat is to be served with the broth, as in the case of a stew, it should be put on in cold water, brought quickly to the boiling point (212° F.), then allowed to simmer (185° F.) until the meat is tender. The cheaper cuts should always be used for soups and stews.

In broiling, baking, or roasting the object is to avoid, as far as possible, the loss of nutritive value from the meat. This is accomplished by subjecting the meat to a high temperature, thus searing the surface as quickly as possible, which causes the albumen to coagulate.

### Digestibility.

Meat is easily digested and well absorbed.

Experiments have shown that raw meat is more readily digested than cooked meat, but lacking in taste and flavor, would soon become unbearable if introduced into the daily dietary.

The digestibility of meat depends upon the length and thickness of the individual fibres, the quantity of fat between the fibres, and the hardness and denseness of connecting tissues. Jessen has found that beef and mutton are digested in the same time. It cannot be denied, however, that the fat of mutton is more difficult of digestion than the fat of beef, owing to the larger quantity of stearic acid present.

The meat of young animals (veal excepted) is more easily digested but less nutritious than the meat of older animals — as the walls of the muscle tubes are more delicate and there is less connective tissues.

## WAYS OF COOKING.

### Beef Balls.

Wipe a small piece steak cut from top of round, and cut in one-fourth inch strips. Lay strips on board and scrape separately, using a silver spoon, with grain of meat first on one side and then on other, to remove soft part of meat, leaving the connective tissue. Form into small balls, handling as lightly as possible. Heat a steel omelet pan, sprinkle with salt, shake constantly while adding balls, and continue shaking until the surface of balls is seared. Arrange on buttered toast and garnish with parsley.

### Broiled Beefsteak.

Wipe a small piece steak cut one inch thick. Heat a wire broiler, put in steak, and place over a clear fire, turning every ten seconds for the first minute that surface may be well seared, thus preventing escape of juices. After the first minute turn occasionally until well cooked on both sides. Cook five minutes if liked rare. Remove to hot serving-dish, spread with soft butter, and sprinkle with salt. The most tender steaks are tenderloin, rump, and sirloin. A tenderloin steak lacks juice and flavor; for this reason it is often served with Beef Extract I. (see p. 86) poured over it. A thick slice of sirloin steak with tenderloin attached is known in our markets as a Porterhouse Steak. A round steak is composed of solid lean meat, rich in juices, and if of right age and taken from second or third cut from top of round, is comparatively tender, and cheaper than either rump or sirloin.

### Pan Broiled Beef Cakes.

Wipe and finely chop two ounces steak from upper part of round, season with salt, and shape in a flat, circular cake, using as little pressure as possible. Heat small omelet pan, rub over with fat, put in meat, and turn as soon as under surface is seared, then turn and sear other side. Cook five minutes, turning occasionally, using a griddle cake turner that surface may not be pierced. Brush over with soft butter and sprinkle with salt.

### Broiled Lamb Chops.

Wipe chops, remove superfluous fat, and place in broiler rubbed over with some of the fat. Follow directions for Broiled Beefsteak (see p. 142). When loin chops are used, remove flank and reserve for soup making. The loin chop contains meat on either side of bone and corresponds to the Porterhouse steak in the beef creature.

#### Pan Broiled French Chop.

Select rib chops, and scrape the bone clean nearly to the lean meat, thus making French chops. Put in a hissing-hot frying-pan rubbed over with fat. Sear on one side, turn and sear other side. Cook six minutes if liked rare, eight minutes if liked well done. Turn often while cooking, using knife and fork, that the surface may not be pierced, as would be liable if fork alone were used. Let stand around edge of frying-pan to brown outside fat. When half cooked, sprinkle with salt. Drain on brown paper, remove to serving-dish, spread with soft butter, sprinkle with salt, and stack around a mound of mashed potato, potato balls, or green peas. Trim each chop bone with a paper frill.

#### Broiled Sweetbread.

Put sweetbread in bowl, cover with cold water, and let stand one hour; drain, remove fat, pipes, and membrane. Cook in boiling salted acidulated water twenty minutes, allowing one-half tablespoon each salt and vinegar to a pair of sweetbreads, then drain again and plunge into cold water.

Sweetbreads cooked in this way are called parboiled sweetbreads. This is the first step taken, no matter in what way sweetbreads are to be prepared.

Remove sweetbread from cold water, dry on a towel, split one-half sweetbread lengthwise, sprinkle with salt and pepper, place on a greased fine wire broiler, and broil over a clear fire. As soon as sweetbread is heated, brush sparingly with melted butter, first on one side, then on other. For serving, spread with soft butter, sprinkle with salt, and garnish with parsley.

### Creamed Sweetbread.

Parboil sweetbread and cut in one-half inch cubes. To one-third cup cubes add one-fourth cup White Sauce made as follows:

Melt one-half tablespoon butter, add three-fourths tablespoon flour, and pour on gradually, while stirring constantly, one-fourth cup milk. Season with salt and few grains pepper. Serve in Croustades of Bread (see p. 99).

### Glazed Sweetbread.

Parboil one-half sweetbread, preferably the heart sweetbread. Place in individual baking-dish, and sprinkle with salt. Dissolve one teaspoon beef extract in one and one-half tablespoons boiling water. Pour one-third mixture over sweetbread, put in hot oven and bake until well glazed, basting three times with remaining mixture. Serve with a border of peas.

### Jellied Sweetbread.

Parboil one-half sweetbread and cut in small dice. Have at one hand one-third cup consommé that will jell when cold. Cover bottom of an individual mould with consommé, set mould in pan of ice water, and when consommé is firm, decorate with cold cooked potato, carrot, and truffle cut in fancy shapes. Cover with consommé, and when firm put in layer of sweetbread and enough consommé to hold cubes together. Decorate sides of mould with cooked vegetables and add more sweetbread and consommé. Chill, remove from mould, and place on lettuce leaf.

Chicken stock may be used in place of consommé by adding gelatin to stiffen.

### Broiled Ham I.

Remove outside layer of fat from small piece of ham, cut one-third inch thick, and soak one-half hour in lukewarm water; drain, wipe, and broil three minutes.

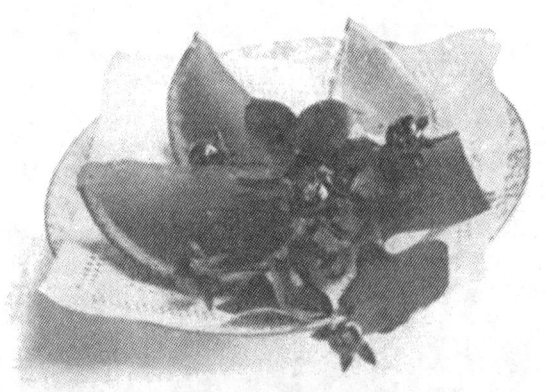

**ORANGE JELLY IN SECTIONS OF ORANGE PEEL**
See p. 180

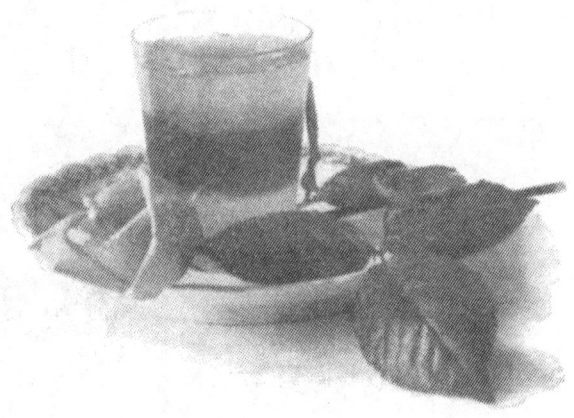

**CHRISTMAS JELLY**
See p. 184

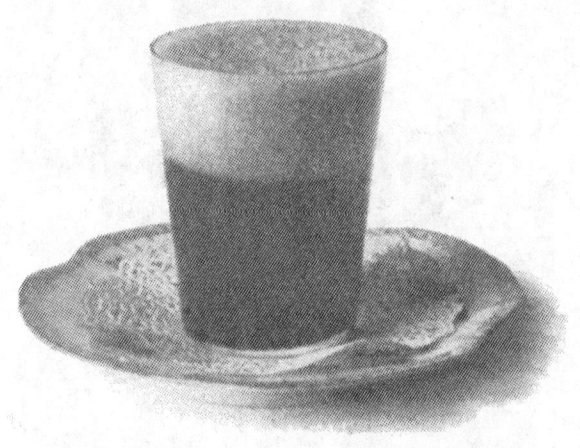

WINE JELLY, MADE TO REPRESENT FRESHLY DRAWN
GLASS OF LAGER BEER

See p. 182

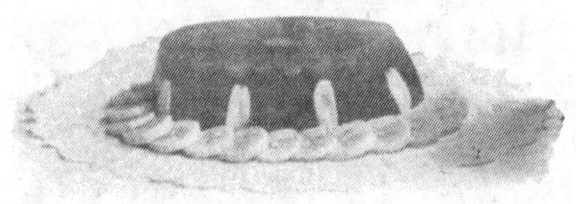

MACEDOINE PUDDING

See p. 186

MEAT. 145

### Broiled Ham II.

Prepare ham as for Broiled Ham I., put in hissing-hot omelet pan, cook one minute on one side, turn and cook one minute on other side. Drain on brown paper and serve at once.

### Bacon.

Cut bacon in as thin slices as possible and remove rind. Place slices closely together in a fine wire broiler, place broiler over dripping-pan, and bake in a hot oven until bacon is crisp and brown, turning once. Drain on brown paper.

### Curled Bacon.

Cut bacon in as thin slices as possible and remove rind. Put slices on board, pass a broad-bladed knife over each slice two or three times, using some pressure, thus making slices still thinner. Put in hot omelet pan one slice at a time, when slices will curl. Cook until brown, then drain.

### Broiled Chicken.

Order chicken split for broiling. Singe, wipe, sprinkle with salt, and place on a well-greased broiler. Broil twenty minutes over a clear fire, watching carefully and turning broiler so that all parts may be browned equally. The flesh side needs the longer exposure to the fire. The skin side cooks quickly and then is liable to burn. Remove to hot platter, spread with soft butter, and sprinkle with salt.

So much time and attention is required for broiling a chicken that the work is often simplified by placing chicken in dripping-pan, skin side down, sprinkling with salt, dotting over with butter, and cooking fifteen minutes in a hot oven, then removing to broiler to finish the cooking.

### Maryland Chicken.

Dress, clean, and disjoint one-half broiler. Sprinkle with salt, dip in flour, egg (slightly beaten and diluted with two tablespoons cold water), and soft stale bread crumbs. Place in a well-greased dripping-pan and bake twenty minutes in a hot oven, basting after first five minutes of cooking with two tablespoons melted butter. Arrange on serving-dish and pour around one-half cup White Sauce made as follows:

Melt one-half tablespoon butter, add one tablespoon flour, and pour on gradually, while stirring constantly, one-half cup thin cream. Season with salt.

### Roast Chicken.

Dress, clean, and truss a small chicken. Place on back on rack in dripping-pan. Rub entire surface with salt, and spread breast and legs with one and one-half tablespoons butter rubbed until creamy and mixed with one and one-half tablespoons flour. Dredge bottom of pan with flour. Place in hot oven, and when flour is well browned, reduce heat, then baste chicken. Continue basting every ten minutes until chicken is cooked. For basting use two tablespoons butter melted in one-half cup boiling water, and after this is gone use fat in pan. During cooking, chicken must be turned frequently, that it may brown evenly. Made gravies are rich, difficult of digestion, and not adapted for invalid cookery; therefore the recipe for the making of gravy is omitted.

### Creamed Chicken.

Cut cold broiled fowl in one-third inch cubes; there should be one-third cup. Add to White Sauce made as follows:

Melt one-half tablespoon butter, add three-fourths tablespoon flour, and pour on gradually, while stirring constantly, one-fourth cup milk. Season with salt, pepper, and celery salt.

MEAT. 147

### Chicken Timbale.

Remove piece of breast meat from an uncooked chicken, chop finely, then force through a fine strainer, using a wooden potato masher; there should be two tablespoons. Pound in mortar, add gradually one-half egg white, and work until smooth. Then add gradually one-fourth cup heavy cream. Season with salt and pepper. Turn into a slightly buttered individual tin mould, set mould in pan of hot water, cover with buttered paper, and bake in a moderate oven twelve minutes, or until firm. Remove from mould and pour around White Sauce.

### Chicken and Rice Cutlets.

Follow recipe for Steamed Rice (see p. 104), using chicken stock in place of water. Half fill slightly buttered cutlet moulds with rice, then fill with chicken forcemeat, using recipe for Chicken Timbale. Set in pan of hot water, cover with buttered paper, and bake in a moderate oven until chicken is firm. Remove from moulds and pour around White Sauce.

### Chicken Soufflé.

Melt one teaspoon butter, add one teaspoon flour, and pour on, gradually, while stirring constantly, one-fourth cup milk; then add one tablespoon soft bread crumbs and one-eighth teaspoon salt and cook one minute. Remove from fire and add one-fourth cup cold cooked chicken finely chopped, and cut and fold in one egg white beaten until stiff. Turn into slightly buttered tin mould, set in pan of hot water, cover with buttered paper, and bake in a moderate oven until firm. Remove from mould and pour around White Sauce.

### Broiled Quail on Toast.

Singe, wipe, and with a sharp pointed knife, beginning at back of neck, make a cut through backbone the entire length of bird. Lay open bird and remove contents. Cut out ribs either side of backbone, remove breastbone, and cross legs. Place on a greased broiler and broil eight to ten minutes over a clear fire. Arrange on buttered toast, spread with butter, sprinkle with salt, and garnish with toast points, cubes of jelly, parsley, and lemon.

### Boned Squab in Paper Case.

Butter sparingly, using a butter brush, one-half sheet foolscap paper. Place a boned bird on lower half of sheet and fold upper part over bird, bringing edges together. Begin at edges and fold over lower side and ends of paper three times. Place in a wire broiler and broil ten minutes over a slow fire, turning often, being careful that paper does not catch on fire. Remove bird from case on to a slice of buttered toast, season with salt and pepper, spread with soft butter, and garnish with toast points, cubes of jelly, lemon, and parsley.

A breast of chicken, tenderloin of steak, or lamb chop may be broiled in a paper case.

### How to bone a Bird.

In buying birds for boning, select those which have been fresh killed, dry picked, and not drawn. Singe, remove pin-feathers, head, and feet, and cut off wings close to body. Lay bird on a board, breast down.

Begin at neck and with sharp knife cut through the skin the entire length of body. Scrape the flesh from backbone until end of one shoulder-blade is found; scrape flesh from shoulder-blade and continue around wing-joint, cutting through tendinous portions which are encountered; then bone other side. Scrape skin from backbone the entire length of body, working across the ribs. Free wishbone and collar-bones, at same time removing crop and windpipe; continue down breastbone, particular care being taken not to break the skin, as it lies very near bone, or to cut the delicate membranes which enclose entrails. Scrape flesh from second joints and drumsticks, laying it back and drawing off as a glove may be drawn from the hand. Withdraw carcass and put flesh back in its original shape.

### Broiled Tenderloin of Beef with Beef Marrow.

Saw a marrow-bone into one and one-fourth inch pieces. Remove marrow and put in boiling salted water. Cook eight minutes, keeping water just below the boiling point. Remove to circular pieces of Broiled Beef Steak. (See p. 142.)

## MEAT AND FISH SAUCES.

### White Sauce I. (For Vegetables.)

½ tablespoon butter. ⅓ cup milk.
⅔ tablespoon flour. Few grains salt.

Melt butter, add flour, and when well mixed pour on gradually, while stirring constantly, milk. Bring to boiling-point, then season.

### White Sauce II. (For Meat and Fish.)

½ tablespoon butter. ⅓ cup milk.
1 tablespoon flour. Salt.

Make same as White Sauce I.

### Egg Sauce I.

To White Sauce I. add one-half "hard boiled" egg thinly sliced or chopped.

### Egg Sauce II.

To White Sauce I. add yolk one egg slightly beaten and a few drops lemon juice.

### Drawn Butter Sauce.

Melt three-fourths tablespoon butter, add three-fourths tablespoon flour, and when well mixed pour on gradually, while stirring constantly, one-half cup boiling water. Season with salt, then add three-fourths tablespoon butter in small pieces, and one-half "hard boiled" egg cut in thin slices.

### Tomato Sauce.

½ tablespoon butter.  ⅓ cup stewed and strained
¾ tablespoon flour.    tomatoes.
                      Few grains salt.
Few grains pepper.

Brown butter, add flour and stir until slightly browned; then pour on gradually, while stirring constantly, tomato. Season with salt and pepper. A few drops onion juice is an improvement to this sauce.

### Béchamel Sauce.

½ tablespoon butter.    ⅓ cup chicken stock and cream
⅔ tablespoon flour.        in equal parts.
                      Few grains salt.

Make same as White Sauce I.

### Yellow Béchamel Sauce.

To Béchamel Sauce add just before serving one egg yolk slightly beaten.

### Maître d'Hôtel Butter.

Cream one tablespoon butter, add gradually one-third teaspoon lemon juice, one-eighth teaspoon salt, a few grains pepper, and one-half teaspoon finely chopped parsley.

# CHAPTER XX.

## VEGETABLES.

### Table showing Composition.

| Article. | Proteid. | Fat. | Carbo-hydrates. | Mineral matter. | Water. | Calorie value per lb. |
|---|---|---|---|---|---|---|
| Asparagus . . . | 1.8 | .2 | 3.3 | 1.0 | 94.0 | 105 |
| Beans, lima, green | 7.1 | .7 | 22.0 | 1.7 | 68.5 | 570 |
| Beans, green string | 2.2 | .4 | 9.4 | 0.7 | 87.3 | 235 |
| Cauliflower . . . | 1.6 | .8 | 6.0 | 0.8 | 90.8 | 175 |
| Celery . . . . | 1.4 | .1 | 3.0 | 1.1 | 94.4 | 85 |
| Lettuce . . . . | 1.3 | .4 | 3.3 | 1.0 | 94.0 | 85 |
| Onions . . . . | 4.4 | .8 | 0.5 | 1.2 | 93.5 | 210 |
| Peas, green . . . | 4.4 | .5 | 16.1 | 0.9 | 78.1 | 400 |
| Potatoes, white . | 2.1 | .1 | 18.0 | 0.9 | 78.9 | 380 |
| Spinach . . . . | 2.1 | .5 | 3.1 | 1 9 | 92.4 | 120 |
| Squash . . . . | 1.6 | .6 | 10 4 | 0 9 | 86.5 | 245 |
| Tomatoes . . . | 0.8 | .4 | 3.9 | 0.5 | 94.4 | 105 |

PROF. W. O. ATWATER.

THE so-called vegetables, with the exception of peas, beans, and lentils, contain a small amount of nutriment, but are valuable, nevertheless, for the large amount of water and the mineral matter they contain. Vegetables are necessary for the body's needs, as they give bulk to the food and possess especial antiscorbutic properties.

In selecting summer vegetables, choose those that are fresh and crisp, and when possible purchase from the producer, as they should be cooked as soon after gathering as possible.

Beans and peas, when fresh, young, and tender, may be used to advantage in the sick-room. If served when old, they should be pressed through a strainer after being cooked, and made into a purée or soup. In this way the cellulose may be discarded.

Asparagus appears in the market as one of the early native vegetables, and may be introduced into the dietary of the convalescent.

In the spring of the year many patients long for dandelions. Their peculiar bitter flavor acts as a stimulant to a flagging appetite. A desire is often expressed for beet greens, which may be indulged.

Cauliflower may be used by the convalescent, while cabbage, which belongs to the same family, should be avoided except by the people who serve it frequently when in health. During the cooking of cabbage certain ferments are developed which cause the vegetable when eaten to give rise to stomach eructations.

Onions are wholesome and quite nutritious to persons with whom they agree. The Bermuda and Spanish onions are much more delicate in flavor than the common garden onion. Onions impart a strong odor to the breath, due to volatile substances absorbed by the blood, and by the blood carried to the lungs, where they are set free.

The use of broiled or stewed tomatoes in many diseases is not objectionable; however, in cases where citric acid is to be avoided, tomatoes must be excluded from the dietary. A reliable brand of canned tomatoes is quite as satisfactory as the fresh vegetable if the canned goods are thoroughly re-oxygenated.

Spinach is found in the market throughout the year, but is especially desirable during the winter, when most of the green vegetables are expensive and of inferior quality.

Among the summer vegetables, green corn and cucumbers should be avoided, as they are the source of much stomach and bowel trouble.

Unless one has access to the large city markets, the supply of vegetables during the winter months is limited to squash, turnips, carrots, parsnips, beets, cabbage, and onions. Squash is the only one among them all that

VEGETABLES. 153

would not be subject to unfavorable criticism if used in the feeding of the sick, and even this vegetable must be excluded from the dietary of the diabetic.

Lettuce is classed among salad greens. It may be obtained usually throughout the year, as it is raised during the winter in hothouses, at which time it is especially palatable. It should be fresh and crisp. The outer leaves, which are usually somewhat wilted, should be discarded. The food value of lettuce is much increased when served with a French Dressing. Many a thin person would find a real fattening agent in olive oil.

The young, tender stalks of celery often prove an appetizer, while radishes would better be avoided on account of the large amount of cellulose they contain.

Among other salad greens may be named chickory, water-cress, romaine, and escarole, all of which may be occasionally introduced into the menu of the convalescent.

### Cooking of.

Vegetables, like all starchy foods, should be cooked in freshly boiling water, salt often being added to give flavor. By the application of hot water the starch grains swell and burst, which gives the starch an opportunity to escape through the layers of cellulose.

From this statement it may be seen that cookery plays a very important part towards the complete digestion of starchy foods.

Vegetables contain such a small quantity of proteid that the loss during cooking should be made as slight as possible. Like animal proteid, it is coagulated by heat. It is more soluble in cold water than animal proteid. Thus if vegetables are allowed to soak in cold water for too long a time, there will be an appreciable loss in nutritive value, mineral matter as well as proteid.

### Digestibility.

The digestibility of vegetables depends upon their bulk and the quantity of cellulose they contain. The cellulose encloses the starch grains, thus making it difficult for the gastric juices to penetrate to the chief constituent of most vegetable foods, — starch.

Neither hot nor cold water has any material effect on cellulose, even in young, tender vegetables. It may be stated as a general rule that vegetable food is less completely digested and absorbed than animal food. There are, however, some striking exceptions to this rule, namely, macaroni and rice.

Vegetables throw a large amount of mechanical work on the stomach. As the gastric ferments play no part in the digestion of starchy foods, and as the food must be reduced to such a consistency as to be able to be forced on into the small intestine, it would seem desirable to restrict this class of foods for those with enfeebled digestion.

## WAYS OF COOKING.

### Boiled Asparagus.

Cut off lower parts of nine stalks asparagus at the point at which they will snap. Wash, remove scales, and tie together. Cook in boiling salted water until soft, time required being from twenty to thirty-five minutes. Tips should be kept out of water for the first ten minutes of the cooking. Drain, place on hot serving-dish, spread with one-half tablespoon butter, and sprinkle with salt.

### Asparagus on Toast.

Serve Boiled Asparagus on buttered toast, moistened with some of the water in which asparagus was cooked.

### Asparagus with Milk Toast.

Serve Boiled Asparagus on Milk Toast, pouring two tablespoons sauce over asparagus.

## VEGETABLES. 155

### Creamed Asparagus Tips.

Wash asparagus stalks, remove scales, and cut in one-inch pieces. Cook in boiling salted water until soft, cooking tips a shorter time than stalks. Drain and add to White Sauce I. (see p. 149).

### String Beans.

Remove strings from beans and snap or cut in one inch pieces. Wash in cold water and cook in boiling water until soft, the time required being from one to three hours. Drain and season with butter and salt. Never buy string beans unless they are fresh and will snap easily. Cook beans in as little water as possible.

### Shell Beans.

Shell beans may be bought either in or out of the shell. Wash beans and cook in boiling water from one to one and one-half hours, adding salt the last half hour of cooking. Cook in sufficiently small quantity of water, that there may be none to drain off when beans are cooked. Season with butter and salt.

Shell beans may be cooked some time before needed and reheated for serving, providing butter has not been added.

### Brussels Sprouts in White Sauce.

Pick over two-thirds cup sprouts, remove wilted leaves, and soak in cold water fifteen minutes. Cook in boiling salted water twenty minutes, or until easily pierced with a skewer. Drain and add to White Sauce I. (see p. 149).

### Creamed Cauliflower.

Remove leaves, cut off stalk, and soak a small cauliflower thirty minutes, head down, in cold water to cover. Cook, head up, twenty minutes, or until soft, in boiling salted water. Drain, separate flowerets, and to two-thirds cup add White Sauce I. (see p. 149).

### Celery.

To prepare celery for table, cut off roots and leaves, separate stalks, wash, scrape, and chill in cold or ice water. By adding a slice of lemon to water, celery is kept white and made crisp. If one end of stalks is curled, celery looks more attractive for serving.

### Curled Celery.

Cut thick stalk celery in two-inch pieces. With a sharp knife, beginning at outside of stalks, make five cuts parallel to each other extending one-third the length of pieces. Make six cuts at right angles to cuts already made. Put pieces in ice water and let stand for several hours, when celery will curl and be found crisp.

### Beet Greens.

Wash thoroughly, scrape roots, and cut off ends. Drain and cook one hour, or until tender, in a small quantity of boiling salted water. Drain again and season with butter, salt, and pepper.

### Dandelions.

Wash thoroughly, remove roots, drain, and cook one hour, or until tender, in boiling salted water. Drain again, season with butter, salt, and pepper, and serve with vinegar.

### Lettuce.

In buying lettuce select small, heavy heads with firm, light-colored centres. Remove leaves from stalk, discarding outer leaves. Wash in cold water, drain, and dry on towel, putting leaves so that water may drop from them. Keep in cold place until serving time.

French Dressing usually accompanies lettuce.

### Boiled Onions.

Put onions in cold water and remove skins, using a vegetable knife, while under water. Put in saucepan, cover with boiling salted water, and boil five minutes; drain, and again cover with boiling salted water. Cook one hour, or until soft but not broken. Drain again, add a small quantity of milk, cook five minutes, and season with butter and salt.

### Green Peas.

Remove peas from pods, cover with cold water, and let stand one-half hour. Skim off undeveloped peas which rise to top and drain remaining peas. Cook until soft in a small quantity of boiling water. There should be but little if any water to drain from peas when they are cooked. If peas have lost much of their natural sweetness they are much improved by a small quantity of sugar. Season with butter and salt.

### Creamed Peas.

Rinse thoroughly one-third cup canned peas, cover with boiling water, boil one minute, and again drain. Add to peas one-half tablespoon butter and cook four minutes. Dredge with one teaspoon flour mixed with one-eighth teaspoon sugar. Add one tablespoon cream, and salt and pepper to taste.

### Croustades of Peas.

Serve Creamed Peas in Croustades of Bread (see p. 99).

### Boiled Spinach.

Remove roots, carefully pick over (discarding wilted leaves), and wash in several waters, to be sure that it is free from sand. If young and tender put in stew pan, heat gradually, and cook twenty-five minutes in its own juices. If old cook in boiling salted water, allowing one-fourth as much water as spinach. Drain, chop, reheat, and season with butter and salt. Garnish with slices of "hard boiled" egg.

The green color of spinach is better retained by cooking in a large quantity of water in an uncovered vessel.

### Steamed Winter Squash.

Cut in pieces, remove seeds and stringy portion, then pare. Place in a strainer and cook thirty minutes, or until soft, over boiling water. Mash and season with butter and salt.

### Sliced Tomatoes.

Wipe and cover with boiling water, let stand one minute, then remove skins. Chill thoroughly and cut in one-third inch slices.

### Stewed Tomatoes.

Wipe, pare, cut in pieces, put in saucepan, and cook slowly twenty minutes, stirring occasionally. Season with butter, salt, and pepper.

### Broiled Tomatoes.

Wipe, cut in halves crosswise, and cut off a thin slice from rounding part of each half. Sprinkle with salt, dip in crumbs, egg, and crumbs again, place in a well-buttered broiler, and broil six to eight minutes.

## CHAPTER XXI.

### POTATOES.

#### COMPOSITION.

Water, 78.9%.  Proteid, 2.1%.
Starch, 18%.  Mineral matter, .9%.
Fat, .1%.

POTATOES are tubers of the plant *Solanum tuberosum*. It may be seen from studying their composition that their food value lies, principally, in the starch which they contain. Being deficient in proteid and fat, they should be used in combination with such foods as eggs, meat, or fish.

Seldom a day passes that potatoes do not appear on the menu of one or more meals, which proves them to be a popular, inexpensive food. If properly cooked they are more easily digested than most of the vegetable foods, as they contain but a comparatively small quantity of cellulose. Their digestibility is increased by being mashed. If they are allowed to enter the stomach in large pieces, as is sometimes the case when boiled potatoes are served, they are liable to cause gastric disturbance.

The method preferred for cooking potatoes when to be served to a young child or convalescent, is baking, in a hot oven, which changes some of the starch to dextrine, thus increasing its digestibility. If baked in an oven at a low temperature, they have no advantage over boiled or steamed potatoes. Potatoes should be served at once after cooking. Warmed-over potatoes, while very palatable to those in health, should be avoided in the dietary of the sick.

Potatoes contain an acrid principle, the greater part of which lies near the skin. For this reason potatoes are usually pared when prepared for boiling. It must be remembered, however, that there is a greater nutritive loss than when cooked with the jackets on. This loss consists largely of the mineral constituent, which may be well supplied by green vegetables.

When new potatoes first appear in the market they are not a desirable food for the sick-room, as the starch is not thoroughly matured.

### Baked Potatoes.

Select smooth, medium-sized potatoes. Wash, using a vegetable brush, and place on a tin plate. Bake in hot oven forty minutes, or until soft. Remove from oven, press between the fingers, and rupture skin. Take from skin, and serve at once with butter and salt, or cream and salt. If allowed to stand they soon become soggy, as the starch reabsorbs moisture.

### Potatoes served in Shell.

Bake two potatoes. Cut a small piece from top of each, and scoop out inside. Mash, add one-half tablespoon butter, salt, pepper, and one tablespoon hot milk; then add white one-half egg beaten stiff. Refill shells, and bake five minutes in a very hot oven.

### Boiled Potatoes.

2 medium-sized potatoes.   Boiling water.
½ tablespoon salt.

Wash and pare potatoes. Drop at once into cold water to prevent discoloration. Let stand thirty minutes or longer. In the spring several hours will do no harm, as the starch in the potato has become to some extent changed to dextrin, which gives a sweet taste. By long soaking the potato upon cooking becomes more mealy.

Drain, cook in a small saucepan of boiling salted water, being sure water covers potatoes, until soft, which may be easily determined by piercing with a skewer or

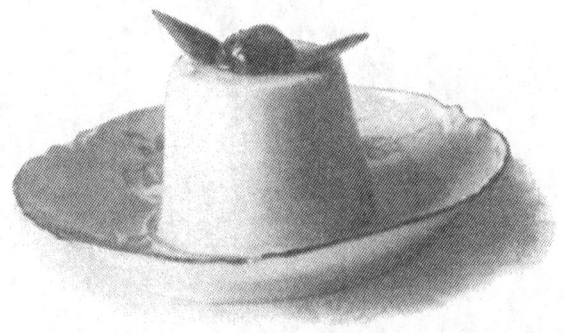

IRISH MOSS BLANC MANGE
See p. 187

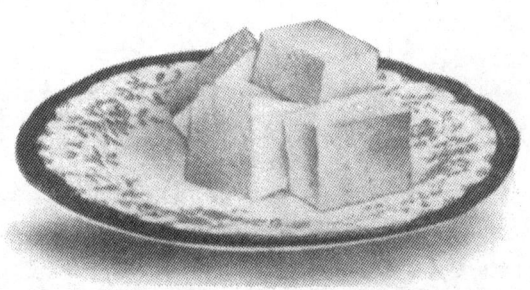

MARSHMALLOW PUDDING
See p. 186

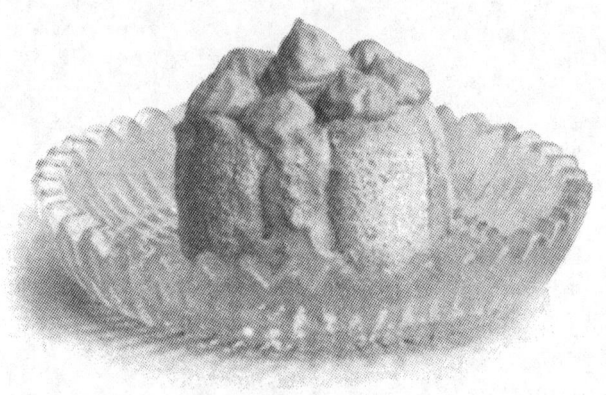

CHARLOTTE RUSSE
See p. 194

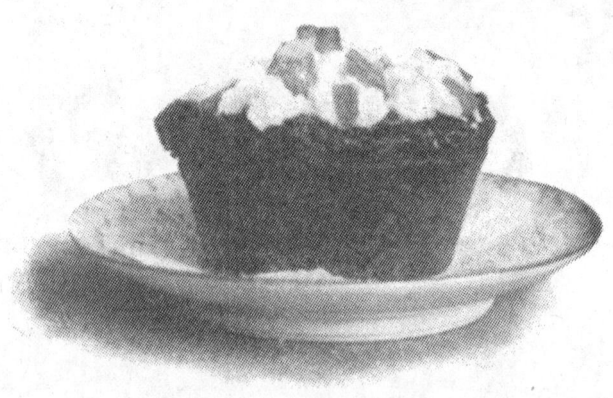

ALMOND TART
See p. 195

fork. Pour off water and let potatoes stand in warm place that steam may escape. Avoid serving in covered dish, as condensed steam causes the potato to become soggy.

### Steamed Potatoes.

Prepare potatoes as for Boiled Potatoes. Put in small strainer, place over kettle of boiling water, cover tightly, and cook until soft.

### Riced Potatoes.

Sprinkle hot Boiled or Steamed Potatoes sparingly with salt, and force through a potato ricer. Pile lightly on serving-dish in form of pyramid.

### Mashed Potatoes. 310 Calories.

To hot Riced Potatoes add one tablespoon butter, hot milk to moisten, and salt to taste. Beat until creamy, using a silver-plated fork. Pile lightly on serving-dish, leaving a rough surface. By smoothing the surface, potato is made compact, and is liable to be soggy.

### Creamed Potatoes.

Wash, pare, and soak potatoes. Cut in one-third inch cubes (there should be one-half cup), and cook in boiling water to cover, to which has been added one teaspoon salt, until soft. Drain, add one-third cup White Sauce, stir lightly with fork to mix potatoes with sauce, and sprinkle with finely chopped parsley.

### Duchess Potato.

Prepare Mashed Potatoes, add yolk one egg, and force through a pastry bag and tube. Serve as a garnish to Broiled Fish.

### Potato Border.

Place a buttered egg cup on small saucer, build around it a wall of hot Mashed Potatoes, and garnish with potato forced through a pastry bag and tube. Remove cup, fill potato border with creamed fish or chicken, and garnish with parsley.

### Potatoes au Gratin.

Prepare Creamed Potatoes, put in buttered baking dish, cover with buttered crumbs, and bake until crumbs are brown. Allow one tablespoon melted butter to one-fourth cup cracker crumbs, and stir with fork until well mixed.

### Potato Balls I.

Wash and pare large smooth potatoes. Shape in balls, using a French vegetable cutter. Soak in cold water and cook in boiling, salted water until soft. Drain, and serve with White Sauce. Sprinkle with finely chopped parsley.

### Potato Balls II.

Prepare same as Potato Balls I., allowing one-half cup, and serve with

Maître d'Hôtel Butter. Cream one tablespoon butter, add gradually one-third teaspoon lemon juice, one-eighth teaspoon salt, a few grains pepper, and one-half teaspoon finely chopped parsley.

## CHAPTER XXII.

### SALADS AND SANDWICHES.

SALADS are compounds of cold cooked meat, fish, eggs, cheese, vegetables, or fruits with a salad green (lettuce, chickory, escarole, romaine, water-cress, cucumbers, celery, or radishes) and a dressing. They find no place in cookery for the sick except during the advanced stages of convalescence, in chronic and wasting diseases, or after a surgical operation.

Salad greens have but little food value, but are useful for the water and potash salts they contain, besides being cooling, refreshing, and stimulating to the appetite. In selecting salad greens choose only those that are fresh and crisp, and see to it that they are thoroughly washed and drained before serving. French dressing greatly increases their nutritive value, and pure olive oil is most beneficial to the system. Cream and Mayonnaise dressings, although highly nutritious, are so complex as to render them difficult of digestion.

Salads are not acceptable unless served cold, and for this reason, especially as they are taken near the close of the meal, they are apt to retard digestion.

Dietitians in hospitals are constantly receiving calls from private wards for salads, and for this reason a few simple salad recipes are introduced. If other combinations are used, avoid vegetables which contain a large quantity of cellulose or many seeds. A lettuce salad served with French dressing is usually the most acceptable one to offer with a dinner. Meat, fish, egg, and cheese salads should furnish the chief dish of a meal, therefore are adapted for luncheon or supper.

## SALAD DRESSINGS.

### Boiled Dressing.

¾ teaspoon salt.
¾ teaspoon mustard.
Few grains cayenne.
1 tablespoon vinegar.
Yolk 1 egg.
1 tablespoon melted butter.
⅓ cup cream.

Mix ingredients in order given, adding vinegar very slowly. Cook over boiling water, stirring constantly, until mixture thickens; strain and cool.

### Cream Dressing I.

½ teaspoon mustard.
½ teaspoon salt.
Few grains cayenne.
¼ cup heavy cream.
1 teaspoon melted butter.
Yolks 2 eggs.
2 tablespoons hot vinegar.

Mix dry ingredients, and add butter, egg, and vinegar. Cook over boiling water, stirring constantly until mixture thickens; cool, and add to heavy cream, beaten stiff.

### Cream Dressing II

3 tablespoons heavy cream.
1 tablespoon vinegar.
⅛ teaspoon salt.
Few grains pepper.

Beat cream until stiff, using smallest size Dover Egg Beater. Add seasonings and vinegar very slowly, continuing the beating.

### French Dressing.

½ tablespoon vinegar.
1 tablespoon olive oil.
⅛ teaspoon salt.
Few grains pepper.

Mix ingredients and stir, using a silver fork, until well blended. French dressing should always be added to salad greens just before serving. If allowed to stand in dressing they will quickly wilt.

## Mayonnaise Dressing.

¼ teaspoon mustard.  
⅓ teaspoon salt.  
¼ teaspoon powdered sugar.  
Few grains cayenne.  
Yolk ½ egg.  
¾ tablespoon lemon juice.  
¼ tablespoon vinegar.  
⅓ cup olive oil.

Mix dry ingredients, add egg yolk, stir until well mixed, and add a few drops vinegar; then add oil gradually at first, drop by drop, and stir constantly. As mixture thickens, thin with vinegar until that is used, then use lemon juice. Add oil alternately with vinegar or lemon juice until all is used, stirring or beating constantly. After the mixture is well thickened the oil may be added in a slow, steady stream, while the beating is continued vigorously. Oil for the making of Mayonnaise should be thoroughly chilled, and egg should be fresh and have been kept in ice box or cold place.

It is desirable, although not absolutely necessary, for bowl containing mixture to be placed in a larger bowl of ice water.

A silver fork, wire whisk, small wooden spoon, or Dover Egg Beater may be used as preferred.

The making of Mayonnaise often troubles the inexperienced cook, while in reality, if the egg is fresh and cold, the oil thoroughly chilled, and the work done quickly and deftly, the process is a very simple one.

During the making of Mayonnaise if the conditions are not right the mixture often becomes curdled. The same thing may take place if too long a time is taken in its preparation. Should it become curdled, a smooth consistency may be restored by taking remaining half of egg yolk and adding mixture slowly to it, beating constantly. A Mayonnaise when done should be stiff enough to hold its shape.

## Oil Dressing.

Yolks 2 "hard-boiled" eggs.  
1 tablespoon olive oil.  
1 tablespoon vinegar.  
¼ teaspoon mustard.  
¼ teaspoon salt.  
Few grains cayenne.

Rub yolks of eggs until smooth, add seasonings, then gradually oil and vinegar.

## SALADS.

### Dressed Lettuce.

Remove leaves from stalk, discarding outside wilted ones. Wash each leaf separately in cold water and shake, holding between thumb and forefinger, that leaves may not be broken. Arrange leaves on a towel in such a way that the water that remains may drop from them. Serve with Boiled or French Dressing.

If the outside leaves are tender, the edges may be trimmed with the scissors, then leaves cut in shreds. Lettuce may be washed, arranged in its original shape, and kept in a covered lard pail in a cool place until needed.

### Egg Salad I.

Cut one "hard-boiled" egg in halves crosswise in such a way that tops of halves are left in small points. To accomplish this a small sharp-pointed vegetable knife is necessary. Remove yolk, rub through a sieve, moisten with Boiled Dressing, and refill whites with mixture. Arrange on lettuce leaves, garnish with thin slices of radish overlapping each other and a radish cut to represent a tulip or chrysanthemum.

How to cut Radishes to represent Tulips. Select smooth, firm red radishes of the round variety. Remove leaves, leaving stems one inch long; beginning at root ends, make seven incisions at equal distances through skin extending nearly to stem ends. Pass knife under sections of skin and cut as far as incisions extend, then make several cuts through fleshy portion. Place in cold water and let stand one hour, when sections of skin will fold back and centres will open.

How to cut Radishes to represent Chrysanthemums. Select round radishes, and cut off a thin slice from the root ends. Scrape radishes in several places to remove some of the red color. Cut from top nearly to stem end in thin parallel slices, then cut thin slices at right angles to slices already cut. Let stand in cold water one hour or more, when radishes will open to look like a flower.

### Egg Salad II.

Separate yolk from white of one "hard-boiled" egg. Finely chop white, moisten with French Dressing, arrange on a lettuce leaf in the form of a circle, and pile yolk, forced through a strainer, in the centre.

### Cheese Salad.

Mash Neufchâtel cheese and shape in form of robin's eggs. Roll in parsley that has been dried in cheese cloth, then very finely chopped. Arrange three eggs on lettuce leaves and serve with French Dressing.

If the cheese crumbles and cannot be readily shaped, moisten with cream.

### Tomato Salad I.

Peel, chill a tomato, and cut in thirds crosswise. Arrange on lettuce leaves and serve with French or Mayonnaise Dressing.

### Tomato Salad II.

Peel a medium-sized tomato, cut a thin slice from stem end, and remove seeds and some of the pulp. Sprinkle inside with salt, invert, and let stand one-half hour. Fill with sweetbread cut in small cubes, mixed with an equal quantity of cold cooked peas and one-half the quantity of finely cut celery moistened with dressing. Arrange on lettuce leaves for serving.

### Tomato Basket with Peas.

Select a small, shapely, bright red tomato, with a piece of the stem left on. Cut in shape of basket, and scoop out pulp and seeds, using a spoon or French vegetable cutter. Refill basket with cold cooked peas moistened with French Dressing and mixed with two halves of walnut meats broken in pieces.

### Chicken Salad.

Cut cold boiled fowl or roast chicken in one-half inch cubes. Wash, scrape, and cut celery in small pieces. Put in bowl of cold or ice water that it may become crisp, then drain and dry on a towel. Just before serving add to chicken, using one-half as much celery as chicken.

Mound on a lettuce leaf, mask with dressing, and garnish with white of egg cut in fancy shapes, yolk of egg forced through a strainer, and capers; or omit lettuce and surround with curled celery.

### Sweetbread and Celery Salad.

Prepare same as Chicken Salad, substituting sweetbread in place of chicken.

A sweetbread and celery salad is attractively served in a ripe red apple prepared by removing a slice from stem end, scooping out all pulp that is possible, leaving just enough that apple may retain its shape.

## SANDWICHES.

The first requisite in the preparation of sandwiches is bread of close, even texture from twenty-four to thirty-six hours old. White, entire wheat, Graham, or brown bread may be used; also Zwieback and some varieties of thin unsweetened crackers. Patients are tempted often to eat bread and butter when served in the form of a sandwich, when they would refuse the slice of bread accompanied by the butter ball. The shape, too, often makes a difference. A heart-shaped sandwich often pleases an adult as well as a child. Men and women are certainly but children of an older growth, which fact is especially emphasized during times of sickness and suffering.

Bread for sandwiches should be cut as thin as possible, and all crusts should be removed. In order to accomplish this a sharp, thin-bladed knife is an essential.

If butter is used it should be creamed (using a wooden spoon or silver fork) and spread on the loaf before the slices are cut, unless the sandwiches are to be formed in round or fancy shapes, when there would be a loss of butter.

After bread is sliced spread one-half the pieces with filling, cover with remaining pieces, and cut in shapes. If bread is first cut in shapes, then one-half the pieces spread with mixture, the mixture either does not come to edges or extends over them, thus detracting from the appearance of the finished sandwich.

If sandwiches are prepared before serving time they may be kept fresh and moist by wrapping in paraffine paper or a napkin wrung as dry as possible out of hot water.

Sandwiches should be served on a plate covered with a doily.

### Bread and Butter Sandwiches.

Remove end slice from loaf of bread, and spread end of loaf evenly with butter which has been creamed.

Cut off as thin a slice as possible, taking care that it is of uniform thickness. Repeat until the required number of slices are prepared. Put together in pairs, remove crusts, and cut in squares, oblongs, or triangles.

### Entire Wheat Sandwiches.

Prepare same as Bread and Butter Sandwiches, using Entire Wheat Bread.

### Raw Beef Sandwiches.

Scrape beef, cut from round, same as for Beef Balls (see p. 141). Prepare bread as for Bread and Butter Sandwiches. Spread one-half the pieces with scraped beef seasoned with salt; if pepper is desired, use sparingly. Cover with remaining pieces, then cut in finger-shaped pieces or triangles.

### Toasted Beef Sandwiches.

Place Raw Beef Sandwiches in a fine wire toaster and place over clear coals or under a gas flame. Brown delicately on one side, turn and brown other side.

### Egg Sandwiches I.

Prepare two slices of bread as for Bread and Butter Sandwiches. Mash yolk of "hard-boiled" egg, using a silver fork, or rub through a sieve. Season with salt and moisten with melted butter or cream, until of the right consistency to spread. Spread on one piece, cover with remaining piece, then cut as desired.

### Egg Sandwiches II.

Finely chop white of "hard-boiled" egg and mix with yolk rubbed through a sieve. Moisten with Boiled Dressing (see p. 164) and spread between pieces of bread prepared as for Bread and Butter Sandwiches.

### Lettuce Sandwiches.

Put fresh, crisp lettuce leaves, washed and thoroughly dried, between thin slices of bread prepared as for Bread and Butter Sandwiches, having a teaspoon of Cream or Mayonnaise Dressing (see pp. 164, 165) on each leaf. The slices of bread must be put together in pairs, cut in shapes, and then separated to insert the lettuce leaf, which should extend over the edge of bread.

### Chicken Sandwiches.

Cut very thin slices from the breast of a cold roast chicken or boiled fowl. Put on slices of buttered bread, sprinkle with salt, cover with slices of buttered bread, and cut as desired.

### Chopped Chicken Sandwiches.

Chop remnants of cold boiled fowl, moisten with rich chicken stock, and season with salt, pepper, and celery salt. Make same as other sandwiches.

### Fig Sandwiches.

Remove stems from figs and chop finely, or force through a meat chopper. Put in double boiler, add a small quantity of water, and cook one hour. Season with lemon juice, cool, and spread between slices of buttered bread.

### Jelly Sandwiches.

Spread Zephyrettes with quince or apple jelly, sprinkle with finely chopped English walnut meat, then cover with Zephyrettes.

### Sweet Sandwiches.

Cut Zwieback (see p. 97), in thin slices, spread with orange or quince marmalade, cover with thin slices of Zwieback, and remove crusts.

## CHAPTER XXIII.

## HOT PUDDINGS AND PUDDING SAUCES.

### Bread and Butter Pudding I.

2 slices stale baker's bread cut ⅓ inch thick.
1 tablespoon butter.
⅔ cup milk.
1 egg.
1 tablespoon sugar.
¼ teaspoon salt.
¼ teaspoon vanilla.

Remove crusts and butter bread, using one-half tablespoon butter for each slice. Put one slice in a buttered baking-dish, pour over milk mixed with egg slightly beaten, sugar, salt, and vanilla, then strained. Cut remaining slice in one-third inch strips and strips in cubes, and put over top. Let stand fifteen minutes. Bake twenty to twenty-five minutes in a moderate oven. Serve with Hard or Creamy Sauce.

### Bread and Butter Pudding II.

Remove crusts from stale bread and force crumbs through a colander; there should be one-fourth cup. To crumbs add two-thirds cup milk, one tablespoon sugar, one-half tablespoon melted butter, one-half beaten egg, and a few grains salt. Turn into a buttered small pudding-dish and bake in a moderate oven. Serve with Lemon or Creamy Sauce I. or II.

### Chocolate Bread Pudding.

Make same as Bread and Butter Pudding II., using one and one-half tablespoons sugar, and adding one-third square melted chocolate. It is best to add sugar to melted chocolate, then pour on gradually the bread and milk mixture before adding butter, egg, and salt.

### Baked Apple Pudding.

⅓ cup stale bread crumbs.
1 tablespoon melted butter.
1½ apples cored, pared, and
   thinly sliced.
1½ tablespoons sugar.
⅛ teaspoon grated nutmeg.
¾ tablespoon water.
⅛ teaspoon salt.

Mix bread crumbs and butter, stirring lightly with fork. Cover bottom of buttered dish with crumbs and spread over one-half the apples. Sprinkle with one-half the sugar, nutmeg, and salt mixed together; repeat and add water. Cover with remaining crumbs, and bake in a moderate oven twenty or twenty-five minutes. Cover at first to prevent pudding browning too rapidly. Serve with Hard Sauce, or sugar and cream.

### Apple Tapioca.

2 tablespoons Minute Tapioca.
⅛ teaspoon salt.
⅔ cup boiling water.
1 apple, pared, cored, and
   cut in eighths.
1 tablespoon sugar.

Mix tapioca and salt and add to boiling water placed on front of range. Boil two minutes, then steam in double boiler fifteen minutes. Butter an individual baking-dish, cover bottom of dish with tapioca, spread over one-half the apples and sprinkle with one-half the sugar; repeat. Cover with remaining tapioca, and bake in a moderate oven until apples are soft. Serve with sugar and cream.

### Peach Tapioca.

Make same as Apple Tapioca, substituting sliced peaches, either canned or fresh, in place of apples.

### Baked Cream of Rice.

1⅔ tablespoons rice.
1¾ tablespoons sugar.
1¼ cups milk.
Few grains salt.
Grated rind ¼ lemon.

Wash rice, add remaining ingredients, turn into a small buttered dish, and bake in a slow oven one and one-half hours. After cooking for fifteen minutes stir to prevent rice from settling.

### Corn Starch Pudding.

⅔ cup scalded milk.  
1½ tablespoons corn starch.  
½ tablespoon sugar.  
⅛ teaspoon salt.  
2 tablespoons cold milk.  
1 egg.  
¼ teaspoon vanilla.

Mix corn starch, sugar, and salt, dilute with cold milk, and add gradually to scalded milk, stirring constantly until mixture thickens. Cover, and let cook in double boiler eight minutes; then add egg slightly beaten, cook one minute, and serve hot with sugar and cream, or mould and chill.

### Chocolate Corn Starch Pudding.

Melt one-third square unsweetened chocolate and add to Corn Starch Pudding before adding egg.

### Tapioca Custard Pudding.

⅔ cup scalded milk.  
1 tablespoon pearl tapioca.  
½ egg slightly beaten.  
1½ tablespoons sugar.  
Few grains salt.  
½ teaspoon butter.

Soak tapioca one hour in cold water to cover, drain, add to milk, and cook in double boiler thirty minutes. Add to remaining ingredients, pour into small buttered baking-dish, and bake about twenty-five minutes in a slow oven.

### Cottage Pudding.

¾ tablespoon butter.  
1½ tablespoons sugar.  
2 teaspoons beaten egg.  
1½ tablespoons milk.  
5 tablespoons flour.  
½ teaspoon baking powder.  
Few grains salt.

Cream butter, add sugar gradually, egg, milk, and flour mixed and sifted with baking powder and salt. Beat vigorously, and turn into two buttered individual tins and bake in a moderate oven. Serve with Creamy, Wine, or Brandy Sauce.

### Chocolate Cottage Pudding.

Make same as Cottage Pudding, adding two teaspoons cocoa with the flour.

### Orange Puffs.

| | |
|---|---|
| 1½ tablespoons butter. | 2 tablespoons milk. |
| ¼ cup sugar. | ½ cup flour. |
| 1 egg yolk. | ¾ teaspoon baking powder. |
| Few grains salt. | |

Make and bake same as Cottage Pudding and serve with

ORANGE SAUCE. Beat the white of an egg until stiff, using a silver fork; add gradually, while beating constantly, one-third cup powdered sugar; then add three tablespoons orange juice, and one-half tablespoon lemon juice.

### Corn Pudding.

| | |
|---|---|
| ⅓ cup scalded milk. | 1 tablespoon brown sugar. |
| ¼ cup popped corn. | ¼ teaspoon butter. |
| ½ egg. | Few grains salt. |

Pick over corn, using the white part only, and roll or pound in mortar until finely divided. Add to milk and butter and let stand until milk is cool; then add sugar, egg slightly beaten, and salt. Turn into a buttered dish and bake in a slow oven until firm, stirring once during baking to prevent corn settling to bottom of dish. Serve with or without cream.

### Custard Soufflé.

| | |
|---|---|
| 1 tablespoon butter. | Yolk 1 egg |
| 1½ tablespoons flour. | White 1 egg. |
| ¼ cup scalded milk. | 1 tablespoon sugar. |
| ⅛ teaspoon vanilla. | |

Melt butter, add flour, and when well mixed pour on gradually milk. Beat yolk of egg until thick and lemon colored, add sugar and continue beating, then add to cooked mixture. Cool and fold in white of egg beaten until stiff and dry and add vanilla. Turn into small buttered dish, set in pan of hot water, and bake until delicately browned and firm. Serve at once, as it will fall if allowed to stand.

### Lemon Soufflé.

Yolk 1 egg.  
¼ cup sugar.  
1 tablespoon lemon juice.  
White 1 egg.

Beat yolk of egg until thick and lemon colored, add sugar gradually, and continue beating, then add lemon juice. Cut and fold in white of egg beaten until stiff and dry. Bake same as Custard Soufflé.

### Fruit Soufflé.

¼ cup fruit pulp, canned peach, or apricot.  
White 1 egg.  
Sugar.

Drain fruit from syrup and rub through a sieve. Heat pulp and sweeten if necessary. Beat white of egg, add gradually hot fruit, and continue beating. Turn into buttered and sugared individual tin moulds, having moulds two-thirds full, and bake same as Custard Soufflé. Remove from moulds and serve with Wine or Lemon Sauce.

### Hard Sauce.

½ tablespoon butter.  
1½ tablespoons powered sugar.  
½ teaspoon sherry or few drops vanilla.

Cream the butter, add sugar gradually, while stirring constantly, then add flavoring.

### Creamy Sauce I.

½ tablespoon butter.  
1½ tablespoons powdered sugar.  
1½ teaspoons milk.  
¾ teaspoon sherry or six drops vanilla.

Cream the butter, add sugar gradually, and milk drop by drop; then add flavoring, drop by drop. The sauce should be of a smooth creamy consistency.

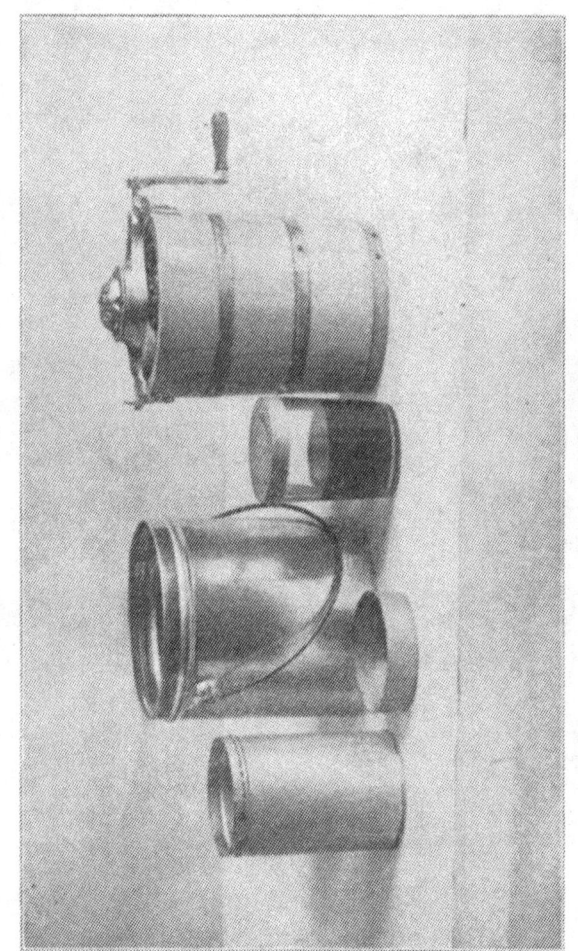

SMALL ICE-CREAM FREEZER AND UTENSILS WHICH MAY BE USED AS SUBSTITUTES

See p. 196

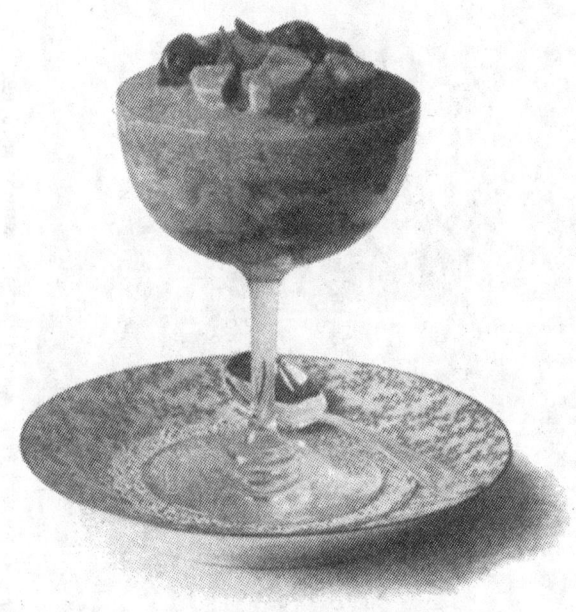

CUP ST. JACQUES
See p. 201

### Creamy Sauce II.

Make same as Creamy Sauce I., using brown sugar in place of powdered sugar.

### Lemon Sauce.

| | |
|---|---|
| 3 tablespoons sugar. | 1 teaspoon butter. |
| ⅓ cup boiling water. | ¾ tablespoon lemon juice. |
| 1 teaspoon corn starch. | Few grains salt. |

Mix sugar and corn starch, add water gradually, while stirring constantly; then let boil five minutes. Remove from fire and add butter, lemon juice, and salt.

### Wine Sauce.

Make same as Lemon Sauce, using one tablespoon Sherry in place of lemon juice.

### Brandy Sauce.

| | |
|---|---|
| ½ egg white. | 3 tablespoons powdered sugar. |
| ½ egg yolk. | Few grains salt. |
| ½ teaspoon brandy. | |

Beat egg white until stiff, and add gradually, while beating constantly, powdered sugar; then add yolk, continuing the beating, and brandy.

### Whipped Cream.

| | |
|---|---|
| 2 tablespoons heavy cream. | Few grains salt. |
| ½ tablespoon powdered sugar. | 4 drops vanilla. |

Put cream in small bowl or cup, add sugar, and beat until stiff, using the smallest size Dover Egg Beater; then add salt and flavoring. Great care must be taken that cream is not overbeaten, which would give it a curdled appearance. Very heavy cream should be diluted with from one-fourth to one-third its bulk of milk.

### Fruit Sauce.

3 tablespoons syrup drained from canned fruit or expressed from fresh fruit.
¼ teaspoon arrowroot.
1 teaspoon cold water.

Heat syrup to boiling point, add arrowroot diluted with cold water, and let boil two minutes.

# CHAPTER XXIV.

## JELLIES.

### Tapioca Jelly I.

2 tablespoons pearl tapioca.  
½ cup cold water.  
⅓ cup boiling water.  
Few grains salt.

Soak tapioca in cold water for several hours or over night; add to boiling water and salt, and cook in double boiler two hours. Serve hot with cream, sherry, and powdered sugar.

### Tapioca Jelly II.

2 tablespoons pearl tapioca.  
½ cup cold water.  
⅓ cup boiling water.  
1 tablespoon sugar.  
1½ tablespoons lemon juice.  
Few grains salt.

Soak tapioca in cold water for several hours or over night, add to boiling water, and cook in double boiler two hours; add lemon juice and sugar. Chill before serving.

### Rice Jelly.

¾ tablespoon rice.  
⅙ cup cold water.  
⅛ cup milk.  
½ egg white.  
Few grains salt.

Soak rice in cold water two hours; drain from water and add to milk. Cook in double boiler one and one-half hours. Strain twice through a fine strainer. Add salt, reheat, and add white of egg beaten stiff. Mould and chill. An inch piece of stick cinnamon may be cooked with rice to give variety. Serve cold with fruit sauce or cream.

### Ivory Jelly I. 115 Calories.

¾ teaspoon granulated gelatin.  2 teaspoons sugar.
1 tablespoon cold milk.  Few grains salt.
⅓ cup scalded milk.  8 drops vanilla.

Soak gelatin in cold, then dissolve in scalded milk; add sugar, salt, and vanilla. Strain into mould and chill.

### Ivory Jelly II.

¾ teaspoon granulated gelatin.  2 tablespoons heavy cream.
½ tablespoon cold water.  ½ tablespoon sugar.
¼ cup scalded milk.  Few grains salt.
⅛ teaspoon vanilla.

Soak gelatin in cold water and dissolve in scalded milk; add sugar, salt, and when cool heavy cream and vanilla. Stir occasionally until mixture begins to thicken; then mould. Serve with sugar and cream.

### Lemon Jelly I. 90 Calories.

¾ teaspoon granulated gelatin.  3 tablespoons boiling water.
1 tablespoon cold water.  2 tablespoons lemon juice.
1½ tablespoons sugar.

Soak gelatin in cold water, add boiling water, and as soon as gelatin is dissolved add sugar and lemon juice. Strain through cheese cloth, mould, and chill.

### Lemon Jelly II.

Make same as Lemon Jelly I. As soon as mixture begins to thicken beat with a small egg-beater until white and frothy; then mould and chill.

### Orange Jelly. 120 Calories.

¾ teaspoon granulated gelatin.  ¼ cup orange juice.
½ tablespoon cold water.  1 teaspoon lemon juice.
1 tablespoon boiling water.  1½ tablespoons sugar.

Cut a circular piece of peel one inch in diameter from the stem end of an orange. Introduce handle of a silver spoon into opening thus made and remove pulp and juice. Strain juice from pulp and use in making jelly. The forefinger of right hand may be of assistance in loosening pulp lying close to skin, which should be discarded, as it is apt to make a cloudy jelly. Proceed same as in making Lemon Jelly. Fill orange with mixture, place in pan, and surround with ice to which a small quantity of water has been added. Be sure that it is well balanced, and watch carefully lest it should be upset by the melting of the ice. As soon as jelly is firm cut lengthwise through skin and jelly in halves, again cut halves lengthwise in quarters. Arrange on serving-dish and garnish with glossy green leaves. Whipped cream may be piled in the centre of dish if desired.

### Orange Baskets with Jelly.

Cut two pieces from each orange, leaving what remains in shape of basket with handle, and remove pulp from basket and pieces. Cut top of basket in points, using scissors, and keep baskets in ice water until ready to serve. Strain juice from pulp and follow recipe for Orange Jelly. Turn into a shallow dish, chill, cut in cubes, and fill baskets. Serve on a bed of crushed ice.

### Orange Jelly with Sections of Orange.

Make Orange Jelly. Cut in cubes, place in the centre of a small dish, and arrange sections of orange to form a border. If the orange is sour sprinkle with powdered sugar.

### Wine Jelly I. 105 Calories.

¾ teaspoon granulated gelatin.  3 tablespoons wine.
½ tablespoon cold water.  1 tablespoon orange juice.
1 tablespoon boiling water.  1 tablespoon lemon juice.
1 tablespoon sugar.

Follow recipe for making Lemon Jelly. Mould and chill.

### Wine Jelly II.

¾ teaspoon granulated gelatin.
½ tablespoon cold water.
1 tablespoon boiling water.
¼ cup sherry or Madeira.
1 tablespoon lemon juice.
1 tablespoon sugar.

Follow recipe for making Lemon Jelly. Reserve two tablespoons; turn remainder into small whiskey glass, and as soon as firm, beat the reserved portion with egg-beater until white and frothy and put on top of jelly. It will suggest a freshly drawn glass of beer.

### Port Jelly I.

¾ teaspoon granulated gelatin.
½ tablespoon cold water.
1 clove.
1 inch piece stick cinnamon.
⅓ cup port wine.
1 teaspoon lemon juice.
½ tablespoon sugar.

Soak gelatin in cold water. Cook clove, cinnamon, and port wine ten minutes in top of double boiler, add gelatin, and as soon as gelatin is dissolved, add lemon juice and sugar. Strain through double cheese cloth, mould, and chill.

### Port Jelly II.

¾ teaspoon granulated gelatin.
½ tablespoon cold water.
1 clove.
1 inch piece stick cinnamon.
1½ teaspoons Breakfast Cocoa.
Few grains salt.
⅓ cup port wine.

Make same as Port Jelly I.; add liquid slowly, as soon as scalded, to cocoa mixed with salt. Cook ten minutes, then strain, mould, and chill.

### Stimulating Jelly.

Make same as Port Jelly II. omitting cocoa and substituting one-half teaspoon beef extract.

## Beef Jelly.

½ lb. beef (lower part of round).  
½ teaspoon granulated gelatin.  
1 teaspoon cold water.  
1½ tablespoons boiling water.  
⅛ teaspoon salt.  
Few grains pepper.

Broil beef and express juice as for Beef Extract. Soak gelatin in cold water and dissolve in boiling water; add to beef juice, with salt and pepper. Strain through double thickness cheese cloth. Mould, chill, and serve the day on which it is prepared. A few grains celery salt may be added to give variety.

## Apricot and Wine Jelly.

¾ teaspoon granulated gelatin.  
½ tablespoon cold water.  
1 tablespoon boiling water.  
2 tablespoons syrup drained from canned apricots.  
2 tablespoons sherry.  
1 teaspoon lemon juice.  
1 tablespoon sugar.

Follow recipe for making jelly. Cover bottom of an individual mould with mixture and let stand until firm. Place on jelly one-half of a canned apricot and add gradually remaining mixture, being careful not to add too much at a time, as it might melt the first layer. Chill, remove from mould, and garnish with whipped cream and candied cherries.

## Cider Jelly.

¾ teaspoon granulated gelatin.  
½ tablespoon cold water.  
1½ tablespoons boiling water.  
½ cup cider.  
Sugar.

Make same as Lemon Jelly I., adding sugar to taste.

## Coffee Jelly. 30 Calories.

¾ teaspoon granulated gelatin.  
½ tablespoon cold water.  
⅓ cup hot coffee infusion.  
½ tablespoon sugar.  
Few grains salt.

Make same as Lemon Jelly I. A fourth teaspoon brandy may be added if desired.

### Sauterne Jelly.

¾ teaspoon granulated gelatin.  ½ cup Sauterne.
½ tablespoon cold water.  1 teaspoon lemon juice.
1 tablespoon boiling water.  ½ tablespoon sugar.

Make same as Lemon Jelly I.

### Christmas Jelly.

Follow recipe for Sauterne Jelly and divide in thirds. Put one-third in a small whiskey glass, let stand until firm, then pour into the glass the second third colored with Leaf Green and chilled sufficiently so as not to melt the lower layer. As soon as the second layer is firm, add the remaining third. Chill, remove from glass, and garnish with small sprigs of holly bearing berries.

### Chicken Jelly.

1½ lb. chicken or  8 peppercorns.
½ of a 3 lb. chicken.  Salt.
2½ cups cold water.

Clean chicken, remove fat and skin, and cut flesh and bone into small pieces. Put into a stewpan with water and peppercorns. Bring slowly to boiling point, remove scum, then cook five or six hours, keeping below boiling point. Strain through double thickness of cheese cloth, season to taste with salt, and let stand until firm. Remove fat, reheat, and turn into individual moulds, when it should again stand. In cooking, the liquid should be reduced to one cup. A sprig of parsley, small stalk of celery, and a bit of bay leaf cooked with chicken gives additional flavor, which is sometimes desirable.

### Veal Jelly.

1½ lbs. of veal cut from loin.  6 peppercorns.
2 cups cold water.  Sprig of parsley.
Salt.

Make same as Chicken Jelly, reducing liquid to one and one-third cups.

## Orange in Surprise.

¼ cup orange juice.
2 teaspoons lemon juice.
2 tablespoons sugar.
Yolk 1 egg.

½ teaspoon granulated gelatin.
¾ teaspoon cold water.
Few grains salt.
Pulp from ½ orange.

Mix first four ingredients and cook until mixture thickens, then add gelatin which has soaked ten minutes in cold water; strain, cool slightly, then add orange pulp, drained from juice. Mould, chill, remove from mould and pour around.

### Orange Sauce.

White of ½ egg.
1 tablespoon powdered sugar.

¾ tablespoon orange juice
½ teaspoon lemon juice.

Beat white of egg until stiff, add sugar, gradually, while beating constantly; then add fruit juices.

### Snow Pudding I.

1 teaspoon granulated gelatin.
1 tablespoon cold water.
½ cup boiling water.

¼ cup sugar.
1½ tablespoons lemon juice.
White 1 egg.

Soak gelatin in cold water and dissolve in boiling water. Add sugar and, as soon as dissolved, lemon juice; strain, and set bowl containing mixture in pan of ice water. Occasionally stir, and when quite thick beat until frothy. Add white of egg, beaten stiff, and continue beating until stiff enough to hold its shape. Mould, or pile by spoonfuls on a glass dish. Serve with Steamed Custard.

### Snow Pudding II.

White 1 egg.
½ teaspoon (scant) granulated gelatin.

¾ tablespoon boiling water.
1 tablespoon powdered sugar.
⅛ teaspoon lemon extract.

Beat white of egg on small plate, using a silver fork, until stiff, add gelatin dissolved in boiling water while beating constantly; then add sugar and flavoring. Pile on a glass dish, chill, and serve with Steamed Custard.

### Fruit Blanc Mange.

½ cup milk.
½ cup water.
1⅓ tablespoons hominy.
½ tablespoon sugar.
⅛ teaspoon salt.
Strawberries.

Scald milk, add water, bring to boiling point, add hominy, gradually, and let boil two minutes; then cook in double boiler two hours. After the first hour and one-half of the cooking add sugar and salt. Mould, chill, and garnish with strawberries and whipped cream.

### Jellied Pears.

¾ teaspoon granulated gelatine.
½ tablespoon cold water.
⅓ cup syrup drained from canned pears.
1 teaspoon ginger syrup.
1 tablespoon sugar.
2 teaspoons lemon juice.
1 canned pear.
Small piece Canton ginger cut in thin slices.

Soak gelatine in cold water and dissolve in syrup drained from pears heated to boiling point; then add ginger syrup, sugar, and lemon juice. Strain, and cool. Cover bottom of small mould with pear cut in pieces and strips of ginger; cover fruit with mixture. When firm add more fruit and mixture; repeat until all is used.

### Macedoine Pudding.

Make fruit or wine jelly mixture. Place small mould in pan of ice water and pour in mixture one-third inch deep; when firm, decorate with a slice of banana from which radiate strips of fig placed seed side down. Cover fruit with jelly mixture by teaspoons. When firm add more fruit and remaining mixture. Chill, remove from mould, and surround with thin slices of banana.

### Marshmallow Pudding.

⅔ teaspoon granulated gelatine.
⅓ cup boiling water.
¼ cup sugar.
White 1 egg.
¼ teaspoon vanilla.
Few grains salt.

Dissolve gelatine in boiling water. Put sugar in bowl, add white of egg, and pour over strained gelatine; then add salt and vanilla. Beat mixture fifteen minutes. Chill and cut in pieces the size and shape of marshmallows. Serve with sugar and cream.

# CHAPTER XXV.

## COLD DESSERTS.

### Irish Moss Blanc Mange. 307 Calories.

⅙ cup Irish moss.  1¾ cups milk.
1½ cups cold water.  ⅓ teaspoon vanilla.
Few grains salt.

Pour cold water over moss and let stand twenty minutes; drain from water; pick over moss, discarding discolored pieces; add to milk, and cook in double boiler ten to fifteen minutes. Milk should be but very slightly thickened; the tendency is to have it overcooked and when chilled the dessert is unpalatable because too stiff. Strain, add salt and vanilla. Strain a second time into small moulds or egg cups previously dipped in cold water. Serve with sugar and cream. Sliced fruit makes an agreeable accompaniment or garnish with a candied cherry and angelica.

### Chocolate Irish Moss Blanc Mange.

⅙ cup Irish moss.  Few grains salt.
1½ cups cold water.  ¾ square Baker's Chocolate.
2 cups milk.  2 tablespoons sugar.
½ teaspoon vanilla.  3 tablespoons boiling water.

Make same as Irish Moss Blanc Mange. Melt chocolate over hot water, add sugar, and gradually boiling water; then pour on slowly the strained mixture. Mould, chill, and serve with sugar and cream.

### Steamed Custard. 357 Calories.

Yolks 2 eggs.  1 cup scalded milk.
1 tablespoon sugar.  1 tablespoon wine, or
Few grains salt.  ¼ teaspoon vanilla.

Beat yolks of eggs slightly, add sugar and salt; stir constantly while adding gradually hot milk. Cook in double boiler, stirring until mixture thickens and a coating is formed on the spoon; strain at once. Chill and flavor.

### Steamed Chocolate Custard. 355 Calories.

2 tablespoons sugar.
⅔ teaspoon corn starch.
½ square Baker's Chocolate, or
1½ tablespoons prepared cocoa.

Few grains salt.
1 cup scalded milk.
Yolk 1 egg.
¼ teaspoon vanilla.

Mix sugar, corn starch, cocoa, and salt. Pour on gradually milk. Cook over hot water eight minutes. Dilute egg yolk slightly beaten with some of the mixture, add to remaining mixture, and cook one minute. Strain, cool, and flavor. If chocolate is used, melt over hot water, add dry ingredients, then gradually hot milk. Strain, cool, and flavor. Serve in glass cups. The white of the egg may be beaten until stiff, sweetened, and piled on top of each custard.

### Steamed Caramel Custard. 463 Calories.

1 cup scalded milk.
Yolks 2 eggs.
3 tablespoons sugar.
Few grains salt.
¼ teaspoon vanilla.

Put sugar in a smooth saucepan, stir constantly over a hot fire until melted and discolored, add to milk, and as soon as sugar is dissolved, add gradually to yolks of eggs slightly beaten, and salt. Cook same as Steamed Custard.

### Steamed Coffee Custard.

1 cup milk.
1 tablespoon ground coffee.
1½ tablespoons sugar.
Yolks 2 eggs.
Few grains salt.
¼ teaspoon vanilla or brandy.

Scald milk with coffee, strain, and make same as Steamed Custard.

### Baked Custard. 273 Calories.

1 egg.
1½ tablespoons sugar.
Few grains salt.
⅔ cup scalded milk.
Few gratings nutmeg, or
Few grains powdered cinnamon.

Beat egg slightly, add sugar and salt. Pour on gradually hot milk, strain into small buttered moulds, sprinkle with nutmeg or cinnamon, set in pan of hot water, and bake in a slow oven until firm. Remove from moulds for serving.

### Baked Purity Custard. 101 Calories.

White 1 egg.
½ tablespoon sugar.
⅓ cup scalded milk.
⅛ teaspoon vanilla.
Few grains salt.

Stir white of egg with silver fork to set free the albumen by breaking the cell walls. Add milk gradually, salt, and flavoring. Strain, and bake same as Baked Custard, the time for cooking being somewhat longer.

### Baked Caramel Custard.

1 egg.
2 tablespoons sugar.
⅔ cup scalded milk.
⅛ teaspoon vanilla.
Few grains salt.

Put sugar in a smooth saucepan, and stir constantly over a hot fire until melted and of the color and consistency of maple syrup. Pour on the hot milk, and as soon as sugar is dissolved add gradually to egg slightly beaten; then add salt and vanilla. Bake same as plain custard. Serve with

CARAMEL SAUCE. — Melt three tablespoons sugar, and as soon as well browned add three tablespoons water. Cook five minutes, then cool slightly.

### Baked Coffee Custard.

⅔ cup milk.  
¾ tablespoon ground coffee.  
Few grains salt.  
1 egg.  
½ teaspoon brandy, or  
⅛ teaspoon vanilla.  
1½ tablespoons sugar.

Scald milk with coffee. Strain, and make same as Baked Custard. Omit flavoring, if desired, as coffee alone would suit the taste of most people.


### Junket Custard.

¾ cup milk.  
1 tablespoon sugar.  
⅔ tablespoon brandy, or  
¼ teaspoon vanilla.  
¼ Junket tablet, or  
1 teaspoon Fairchild's essence Pepsin.  
1 teaspoon cold water.  
Few grains salt.

Heat milk until lukewarm, add sugar, salt, flavoring, and tablet dissolved in cold water. Pour quickly into small moulds, let stand in a warm place until set, then put in cold place to chill. Remove from moulds, and serve with or without sugar and cream. If needed in a hurry, use double the amount of tablet. Sugar may be omitted if desired.


### Caramel Junket.

¾ cup milk.  
1½ tablespoons sugar.  
Few grains salt.  
2 tablespoons boiling water.  
¼ Junket tablet, or  
1 teaspoon Fairchild's essence Pepsin.  
1 teaspoon cold water.  
¼ teaspoon vanilla.

Heat milk until lukewarm. Caramelize sugar, add boiling water, and cook until reduced to one tablespoon. Add to milk, and when well mixed add tablet dissolved in cold water and vanilla. Mould, chill, and serve.

## COLD DESSERTS.

### Tapioca Cream I.

1½ tablespoons Minute Tapioca.
⅓ cup scalded milk.
2 teaspoons sugar.
Few grains salt.
¼ egg white.
6 drops vanilla.

Cook tapioca and milk in double boiler thirty minutes, then add sugar and salt; remove from range, add white of egg beaten until stiff, and vanilla. Chill, and serve with cream, cooked fruit, or fruit sauce.

### Tapioca Cream II.

¾ tablespoon Minute Tapioca.
⅔ cup scalded milk.
2 tablespoons sugar.
Few grains salt.
1 egg.
¼ teaspoon (scant) vanilla.

Add tapioca to milk, and cook in double boiler until tapioca is transparent, then add one-half the sugar, and as soon as dissolved pour hot mixture slowly on to remaining sugar mixed with salt, and egg yolk slightly beaten. Return to double boiler and cook until mixture thickens, then add white of egg beaten stiff. Chill and flavor.

### Tapioca with Cocoa.

1 tablespoon Minute Tapioca.
⅓ cup milk.
1 teaspoon Breakfast Cocoa.
¼ egg white.
2 teaspoons sugar.
Few grains salt.
6 drops vanilla.

Cook tapioca and milk in double boiler thirty minutes, then add cocoa, sugar, and salt mixed together. Remove from range and add white of egg beaten until stiff, and vanilla. Mould and chill. Serve with sugar and cream.

### Tapioca with Coffee.

2 tablespoons Minute Tapioca.
⅓ cup filtered coffee.
2 teaspoons sugar.
¼ teaspoon vanilla.

Cook tapioca and coffee in double boiler thirty minutes, then add sugar and vanilla. Mould, chill, and serve with sugar and cream.

### Hamburg Cream.

Yolk 1 egg.
1 tablespoon sugar.
White 1 egg.
1½ tablespoons lemon juice
Few grains salt.

Beat yolk of egg slightly, add sugar, lemon juice, and salt, then cook over hot water until mixture thickens slightly; then add white of egg beaten until stiff. Turn in a glass and chill. Serve with Lady Fingers.

### Orange Cream.

Yolk 1 egg.
¾ tablespoon sugar.
2½ tablespoons orange juice.
1 teaspoon lemon juice.
Few grains salt.
White 1 egg.

Make same as Hamburg Cream.

### Wine Cream. 131 Calories.

Yolk 1 egg.
¾ tablespoon sugar.
White 1 egg.
2 tablespoons wine (sherry or Madeira).
Few grains salt.

Make same as Hamburg Cream.

### Prune Soufflé.

1 cup prunes.
⅓ cup sugar.
Few grains salt.
White 1 egg.
Lemon juice.

Wash prunes, and soak several hours in cold water to cover. Cook in same water until soft, when water should be evaporated. Remove stones, using silver knife and fork, and force pulp through a sieve. Add sugar and lemon juice to taste, and reheat to dissolve sugar, then cool mixture. Beat white of egg until stiff, and add gradually, while beating constantly, three tablespoons prune mixture. Pile lightly on a buttered dish and bake in a slow oven eight to ten minutes. Serve cold with Steamed Custard.

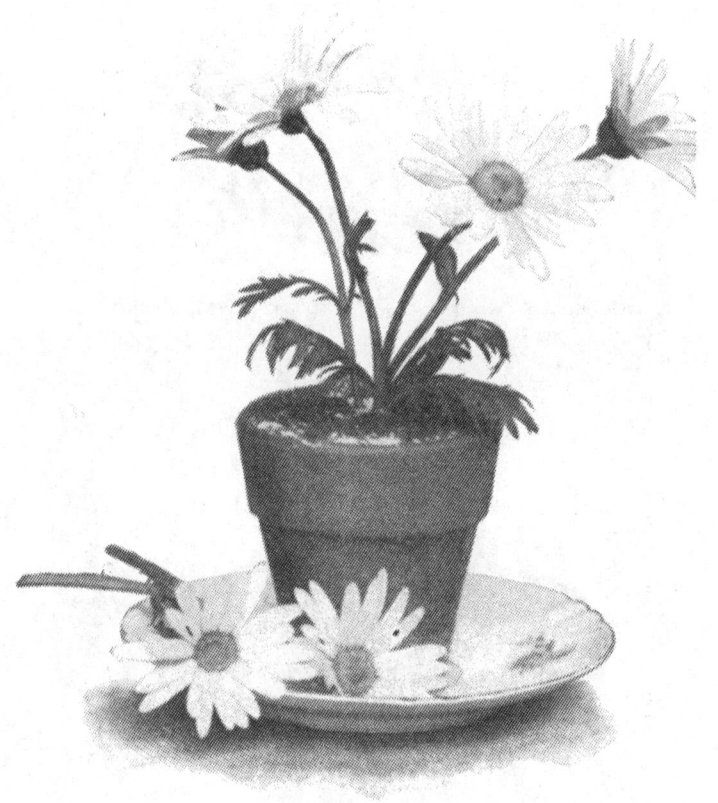

**FLOWERING ICE-CREAM**
See p. 201

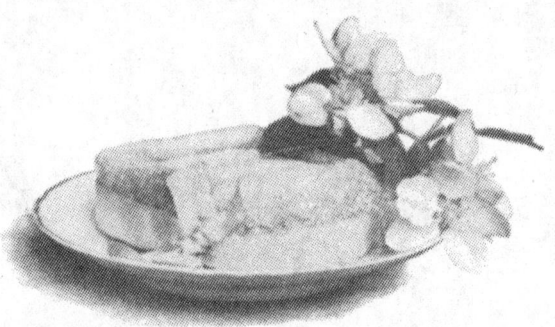

**ICE-CREAM IN A BOX, GARNISHED WITH PINK RIBBON AND APPLE BLOSSOMS**
See p. 201

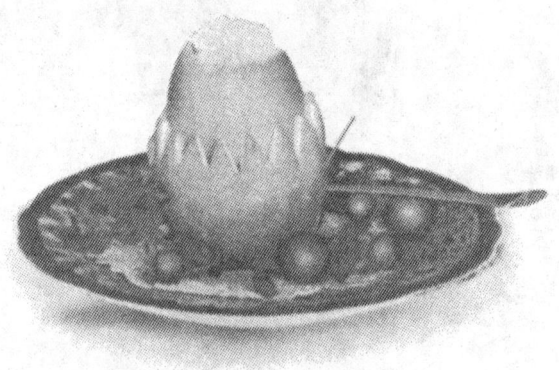

FROZEN EGG CUSTARD
See p. 202

## Spanish Cream.

½ teaspoon granulated gelatin.
½ cup milk.
1 tablespoon sugar.
½ egg yolk.
Few grains salt.
½ egg white.
6 drops vanilla.

Scald milk with gelatin, add sugar, and pour slowly on egg yolk slightly beaten. Return to double boiler and cook until mixture thickens, slightly stirring constantly. Add salt, white of egg beaten stiff, and flavoring. Turn into individual moulds first dipped in cold water, chill, unmould, and serve with sugar and cream.

## Coffee Spanish Cream. 230 Calories.

¼ cup milk.
½ cup coffee infusion.
1 teaspoon granulated gelatin.
2 tablespoons sugar.
Yolk 1 egg.
Few grains salt.
White 1 egg.
⅛ teaspoon vanilla.

Scald milk, add coffee infusion, and gelatin. As soon as gelatin is dissolved, add yolk of egg, beaten slightly, mixed with sugar and salt. Cook over hot water, stirring constantly until slightly thickened; then add white of egg beaten stiff, and vanilla. Turn into individual moulds, first dipped in cold water. Chill, remove from moulds, and serve with sugar and cream.

## Cocoa Cream.

1 teaspoon Breakfast Cocoa.
1 tablespoon sugar.
Few grains salt.
⅓ cup boiling water.
½ cup milk.
1 teaspoon granulated gelatin.
Yolk 1 egg.
White 1 egg.
¼ teaspoon vanilla.

Mix cocoa, sugar, and salt; add gradually, while stirring constantly, boiling water. Let boil one minute, then add milk, gelatin, and as soon as scalded add slowly to the yolk of egg slightly beaten. Cook over hot water until mixture thickens, strain, set in pan of ice water, stir occasionally, and when quite thick, add white of egg beaten until stiff, and vanilla. Mould, chill, and serve with sugar and cream.

### Charlotte Russe. 205 Calories.

¼ cup heavy cream.
⅛ teaspoon granulated gelatin.
½ tablespoon boiling water.
1¼ tablespoons powdered sugar.
Few grains salt.
¼ teaspoon vanilla.
2 Lady Fingers.

Add sugar to cream and beat until stiff, care being taken that cream does not separate. Dissolve gelatin in boiling water, strain through cheese cloth, and add gradually to first mixture; then add salt and vanilla and stir until well mixed. Line mould with Lady Fingers, turn in mixture, chill, and remove from mould for serving.

### Caramel Charlotte Russe.

¼ cup heavy cream.
2 tablespoons sugar.
3 tablespoons boiling water.
⅛ teaspoon granulated gelatin.
½ tablespoon boiling water.
Few grains salt.
⅛ teaspoon vanilla.
2 Lady Fingers.

Put sugar in small omelet pan, place on hot part of range, and stir constantly until melted, and somewhat darker in color than maple syrup. Add boiling water, and let simmer until syrup is reduced to one tablespoon. Add to cream, and beat until stiff. Then add gelatin dissolved in boiling water, salt, and vanilla. Line mould with Lady Fingers, turn in mixture, chill, and remove from mould for serving.

### Chocolate Charlotte Russe.

½ tablespoon Breakfast Cocoa.
1¾ tablespoons sugar.
Few grains salt.
2 tablespoons boiling water.
¼ cup heavy cream.
⅛ teaspoon granulated gelatin.
½ tablespoon boiling water.
⅛ teaspoon vanilla.
2 Lady Fingers.

Mix cocoa, sugar, and salt, add boiling water gradually, and let boil one minute. Cool slightly, add cream, salt,

# COLD DESSERTS. 195

and vanilla, and beat until stiff, then add gelatin dissolved in boiling water and strained. Line mould with Lady Fingers, turn in mixture, and chill.

### Strawberry Charlotte.

Cut selected sweet strawberries in halves lengthwise. Line small mould with berries, turn in Charlotte Russe mixture, chill, and remove from mould for serving.

### Coffee Charlotte Russe.

Make same as Charlotte Russe, adding one tablespoon coffee extract to cream before whipping.

### Almond Tarts.

Yolks 2 eggs.
½ cup powdered sugar.
Whites 2 eggs.
3 tablespoons grated chocolate.
¼ cup Jordan almonds blanched and finely chopped.
½ teaspoon baking powder.
⅓ cup cracker rolled and put through a fine sieve.
Few grains salt.

Beat yolks of eggs until thick and lemon colored, and add sugar, gradually; then fold in whites of eggs beaten until stiff and dry. Add remaining ingredients, and bake in buttered tin gem pans. Cool, remove centres, and fill with whipped cream sweetened and flavored. Garnish with whipped cream forced through pastry bag and tube, and angelica.

### Baked French Custard.

Whites 2 eggs.
1 tablespoon sugar.
Few grains salt.
¼ teaspoon vanilla.
1 cup cream.

Beat eggs until stiff, add gradually sugar and continue the beating; then add salt and vanilla. Scald cream, add egg mixture, and beat with egg beater. Turn into buttered cups and bake until firm. Serve cold with sugar and cream.

## CHAPTER XXVI.

### FROZEN DESSERTS.

FROZEN desserts, whether in the form of ices or creams, are of inestimable value in the sick-room, if given at the proper time and under favorable conditions. They had better be served with a simple meal or between meals, for if introduced as the last course of a dinner they are apt to reduce the temperature of the stomach contents and thus for a time retard digestion. However, if eaten slowly, as they always should be, the effect upon digestion is slighter than is usually supposed.

If eggs and cream enter into their composition, especially if the cream be of good quality, they have a high food value. Patients, especially children, with but little appetite are often tempted by ice cream, and it is frequently ordered by physicians, as they realize the necessity of sufficient nourishment and know the value of the dish they are recommending.

When ice cream is home-made, care must be taken that it is not too rich nor too sweet; there is seldom danger of these errors in the caterer's products.

For the individual recipes of ices and ice creams an ice cream freezer of ordinary capacity proves impracticable. A baby ice cream freezer is on the market which answers the purpose, but as these are owned by but a few, a freezer may be improvised which does the work to the satisfaction of the nurse. A five-pound lard pail, one-pound baking powder can, silver-plated knife and spoon, complete the outfit. If the mixture to be frozen is a water ice, containing fruit juices, a jelly tumbler with fitted cover is substituted for the baking powder can, as the action of the acid on the tin is liable to produce a poisonous compound.

### Chemistry of freezing Ices and Creams.

Ice and rock or coarse fine salt are used for freezing ices and creams. Salt has a great affinity for water, causing the ice to melt rapidly, thus withdrawing heat from the contents of the can, which causes the mixture to freeze. The principle of latent heat is here demonstrated. In the one case the ice, a solid, is changed to a liquid; in the other case the liquid mixture is changed to a solid.

### How to freeze Ices and Creams.

Finely crushed ice and rock or coarse fine salt are necessary for the freezing of ices and creams. They are used in the proportion of three parts ice to one part salt. These proportions are satisfactory for the production of a smooth, fine-grained cream.

If more salt is employed the cream is coarser and less smooth in texture; where less salt is used more time is required for the freezing, with no better results. When water ices are to be frozen, one-half salt and one-half ice is employed, if a granular consistency is desired, as is the case in frappés or granites.

Cover bottom of pail with crushed ice, put in baking powder box or tumbler containing mixture to be frozen, and surround with ice and salt in correct proportions, adding ice and salt alternately, until the pail is two-thirds full.

Turn box or tumbler with hand, and as soon as mixture begins to freeze scrape frozen portion from sides of box or tumbler and beat mixture with a spoon, so continuing until the entire mixture is frozen.

If the baby ice cream freezer is used, fill tub with ice and salt in correct proportions, turn crank slowly at first, that the contents nearest the can may be acted upon by the salt and ice. After the mixture is frozen to the consistency of a mush, then the crank may be turned more rapidly. Do not draw off the water until the freezing is accomplished, unless there is a possibility of the salt water getting into the can.

An ice shaver or a small burlap bag and wooden mallet are the best utensils for crushing ice.

### Lemon Ice.

¼ cup sugar.         ½ cup boiling water.
2 tablespoons lemon juice.

Make a syrup by boiling sugar and water five minutes. Cool, add lemon juice, strain, and freeze, using three parts finely crushed ice to one part rock salt. Serve in frappé or champagne glass.

### Orange Ice.

¼ cup sugar.         ⅓ cup orange juice.
½ cup boiling water.     ½ tablespoon lemon juice.

Make syrup by boiling sugar and water five minutes. Cool, add fruit juices, strain, and freeze. To obtain orange juice, cut orange in halves crosswise, remove pulp and juice, using a spoon, then strain through cheese cloth. A glass lemon squeezer may be used if care is taken not to break the peel. Take out all tough portions and remaining pulp from peel and point tops, using sharp scissors. Fill cups thus made with ice for serving.

### Grape Fruit Ice.

⅓ cup sugar.         ½ cup boiling water.
¼ cup grape fruit juice.

Make same as Orange Ice. Serve in sections of grape fruit pulp. Garnish with candied cherries.

### Pineapple Ice.

⅓ cup canned shredded    ¼ cup cold water.
   pineapple.                Lemon juice.

Add water to pineapple, cover, and let stand in cold place thirty minutes. Strain through cheese cloth, add lemon juice to taste, then freeze. If fresh pineapple is used, add syrup to sweeten.

### Raspberry Ice.

3 tablespoons sugar.    ⅓ cup water.
1 cup raspberries.    1 teaspoon lemon juice.

Sprinkle raspberries with sugar, cover, and let stand one hour; then mash and squeeze through cheese cloth to express as much juice as possible. Add lemon juice and freeze. Raspberry ice made in this way is of a much brighter color than when the fruit juice is added to a syrup.

### Strawberry Ice.

Make same as Raspberry Ice, using strawberries in place of raspberries. The quantity of sugar must depend somewhat on the acidity of the fruit.

### Grape Sherbet.

⅓ cup water.    1 tablespoon orange
2 tablespoons sugar.    juice.
¼ cup unfermented grape    1 teaspoon lemon juice.
  juice.

Mix ingredients in order given, strain, freeze, and serve in frappé glass.

### Milk Sherbet.

½ cup milk.    1 tablespoon sugar.
2 tablespoons lemon juice.

Add lemon juice to sugar and pour on gradually milk; then freeze. One-half milk and one-half cream may be used in place of all milk.

### Vanilla Ice Cream.

½ cup thin cream, or    1 tablespoon sugar.
¼ cup heavy cream and    ½ teaspoon vanilla.
¼ cup milk.    Few grains salt.

Mix ingredients and freeze.

### Pistachio Ice Cream.

Color Vanilla Ice Cream mixture with Burnett's Leaf Green and add one-sixth teaspoon almond extract; then freeze.

### Macaroon Ice Cream.

Roll or pound macaroon drops or stale macaroons; there should be two tablespoons. Add to Vanilla Ice Cream mixture, let stand one-half hour; then freeze.

### Caramel Ice Cream.

| | |
|---|---|
| 1/3 cup thin cream, or | 1½ tablespoons sugar. |
| 1/6 cup milk and | 1 tablespoon boiling water. |
| 1/6 cup heavy cream. | 1/3 teaspoon vanilla. |
| Few grains salt. | |

Put sugar in a small saucepan; place on range and stir constantly until melted. Add water, and boil until mixture is reduced to one tablespoon. Add cream very slowly, vanilla, and salt; then freeze.

### Coffee Ice Cream.

| | |
|---|---|
| 1 tablespoon ground coffee. | ¼ cup heavy cream. |
| ¼ cup milk. | 1 tablespoon sugar. |
| Few grains salt. | |

Add coffee to milk, cook over hot water five minutes, and strain. Add remaining ingredients, strain through cheese cloth, and freeze.

### Chocolate Ice Cream.

| | |
|---|---|
| ¼ square Baker's Chocolate. | 1/3 cup thin cream. |
| 1 tablespoon sugar. | Few grains salt. |
| 1 tablespoon boiling water. | 10 drops vanilla. |

Melt chocolate in small saucepan placed over hot water, add sugar and boiling water gradually, stirring constantly. Pour on slowly cream, add salt and vanilla, then freeze.

### Concord Ice Cream.

5 tablespoons thin cream.
1½ tablespoons heavy cream.
1 tablespoon sugar.
4 tablespoons unfermented grape juice.
Lemon juice.

Mix cream, sugar, and grape juice, then add lemon juice to taste, and freeze.

### Frozen Chocolate with Whipped Cream.

½ cup milk.
⅓ square Baker's Chocolate.
1¾ tablespoons sugar.
2½ tablespoons boiling water.
Few grains salt.

Scald milk, and add one tablespoonful sugar. Melt chocolate, add remaining sugar, salt, and, gradually, boiling water. Let boil one minute, add gradually scalded milk, cool, freeze, and serve in frappé glass with Whipped Cream (see p. 177).

### Cup St. Jacques.

Fill champagne glass one-half full of Lemon, Orange, or Strawberry Ice. Make depression in centre, and pour in three-fourths teaspoon Maraschino cordial. Fill glass, slightly rounding with ice, and garnish with banana cut in one-fourth inch slices and slices cut in quarters, candied cherries cut in halves, and Malaga grapes from which skin and seeds have been removed. If Strawberry Ice is used, garnish with banana, and strawberries cut in halves.

### Flowering Ice Cream.

Line a flower-pot, having a two and one-half inch diameter at top, with paraffine paper, fill with ice cream, and sprinkle with grated vanilla chocolate to represent earth. Insert a flower in the centre of cream.

### Ice Cream in a Box.

Trim four Lady Fingers on ends and one edge, so that when put together they will make a square. Put on serving plate and tie in place with narrow ribbon. Insert in box thus made a slice from a small brick of ice cream. Garnish with flowers and serve. If apple blossoms are employed, use pink ribbon; if buttercups, yellow ribbon; if violets, lavender ribbon. Pieces of ice cream may be bought for ten cents at many restaurants and caterers, of correct size for the Lady Finger box.

### Frozen Egg Custard.

Beat yolk of one egg until thick, add, gradually, two tablespoons sugar, few grains salt, one and one-half tablespoons brandy and one-half cup rich milk. Beat white of one egg until stiff, add to first mixture, then freeze. Serve in egg shell placed in lemon cup.

## CHAPTER XXVII.

## FRUITS AND HOW TO SERVE THEM.

### COMPOSITION.

| Fresh Fruits. | Refuse. Per cent. | Water. | Proteid. | Fat. | Carbohydrates. | Ash. | Fuel value per pound. Calories. |
|---|---|---|---|---|---|---|---|
| Apples, | 25.0 | 63.3 | .3 | .3 | 10.8 | .3 | 220 |
| Apricots, | 6.0 | 79.9 | 1.0 | | 12.6 | .5 | 225 |
| Bananas, | 35.0 | 48.9 | .8 | .4 | 14.3 | .6 | 300 |
| Cranberrries, | | 88.9 | .4 | .6 | 9.9 | .2 | 215 |
| Grapes, | 25 0 | 58.0 | 1.0 | 1.2 | 14 4 | .4 | 335 |
| Lemons, | 30 0 | 62.5 | .7 | .5 | 5.9 | .4 | 145 |
| Oranges, | 27.0 | 63 4 | .6 | .1 | 8.5 | .4 | 170 |
| Mushmelons, | 50.0 | 44.8 | .3 | | 4.6 | .3 | 90 |
| Pineapples (edible portion), | | 89.3 | .4 | .3 | 9.7 | .3 | 200 |
| Plums, | 5.0 | 74.5 | .9 | | 19.1 | .5 | 370 |
| Raspberries (red), | | 85.8 | 1.0 | | 12.6 | .6 | 255 |
| Strawberries, | 5.0 | 85.9 | .9 | .6 | 7.0 | .6 | 175 |
| Dried Fruits. | | | | | | | |
| Dates, | 10.0 | 13.8 | 1.9 | 2.5 | 70.6 | 1.2 | 1450 |
| Figs, | | 18.8 | 4.3 | .3 | 74.2 | 2.4 | 1475 |
| Prunes, | 15.0 | 19.0 | 1.8 | | 62.2 | 2 0 | 1190 |

FRUITS are, usually, at their best when served fresh, ripe, and in season, and there are but few with whom they do not agree. Those who cannot take them in the raw state often find them acceptable when cooked.

Fresh fruits have but little food value, but their use in dietaries is of great importance nevertheless, on account of the mineral constituents which they contain. These constituents are made of potash combined with various vegetable acids, namely, tartaric, citric, malic, oxalic, etc., which render the blood more alkaline and the urine less acid. The antiscorbutic value of fruits is due to these constituents. A case of scurvy is quickly acted upon by the use of fresh fruits.

The nutritive value of fruits is chiefly in the form of fruit sugar (levulose), although some fruits contain cane sugar (sucrose) as well as fruit sugar. Examples: apples, apricots, pineapples, etc. The carbohydrate of fruit contains, besides sugar, vegetable gums, which when boiled yield a jelly-like substance. Exception must be made to bananas, which contain their carbohydrate largely in the form of starch. Dried fruits have much greater nutritive value than fresh fruits. Weight for weight, dried figs are more nourishing than bread.

The flavor of fruits, although of no nutritive value, helps to make them useful as foods, as they act as stimulants to the appetite and aids to digestion.

In selecting fresh fruit choose that which is sound, firm, and not over-ripe. Fruit which has began to decompose contains micro-organisms, which are likely to cause many ills. Bruised, imperfect fruit, even if bought at a small price, proves no economy.

### Cooking of.

The flavor of fruits is impaired by cooking, but when they contain a large proportion of cellulose their digestibility is increased.

Cooking fruits also converts their gums into a gelatinous form, which change is demonstrated in the making of jellies.

Unripe fruits, which ought never to be allowed in the raw state, are rendered fit for consumption by cooking.

### Digestibility.

The digestibility of fruits depends largely upon the quantity of cellulose they contain, their number of seeds, and their ripeness; also the fineness of their division when reaching the stomach.

Peach pulp forced through a sieve or scraped apple pulp is often easily digested, when, if eaten in the usual way and imperfectly masticated, would prove a stomach irritant. When unripe fruits are eaten their excess of acids causes pain, colic, diarrhœa, and nausea. During the ripening of fruits their sugar increases, while their acids decrease. Ripe fruits act as a mild stimulant to digestion.

### Baked Apples.

Wipe, core, and pare sour apples. Put in an earthen or granite ware baking-dish, fill cavities with sugar, and allow six drops lemon juice to each apple, then cover bottom of dish with boiling water. Bake in a hot oven until soft, basting every eight minutes with syrup in dish. Care must be taken that apples do not lose their shape. In the spring of the year when apples are somewhat flat and insipid to the taste, a few gratings nutmeg, which should be mixed with the sugar, are a great improvement to baked apples. Serve hot or cold, with or without sugar and cream.

### Apple Sauce.

Wipe, quarter, core, and pare two apples. Make a syrup by boiling one-third cup, each, water and sugar, and a few grains salt, six minutes. Add apple to cover bottom of saucepan, and cook until soft, watching carefully that sections of apple do not lose their shape. Remove from syrup, then cook remaining pieces. Strain syrup remaining in pan over apples.

### Strained Apple Sauce.

Wipe, quarter, core, and pare one and one-half apples. Put in saucepan, sprinkle with sugar, add a few grains salt, and enough water to prevent apples from burning. Cook slowly until apples are soft, then rub through a sieve.

The quantity of sugar and water used must depend on the sweetness and juiciness of the fruit.

### Baked Apple Sauce.

1½ apples (pared, cored, and cut in eighths).  
2 tablespoons brown sugar.  
1 teaspoon lemon juice.  
1 tablespoon water.

Put alternate layers of apple, sugar, and seasonings in a small earthen baking-dish; cover, and bake in a slow oven for one hour. A few gratings nutmeg may be used if desired. Serve hot or cold.

### Apples in Bloom.

Select a medium-sized bright red apple. Wipe, and put in small saucepan. Add two-thirds cup boiling water and cook slowly until apple is soft, turning frequently. Take from saucepan, and remove skin carefully, using a silver knife. Scrape off all pulp that adheres to skin and replace on apple, that the red color may not be lost. To water in saucepan add one and one-half tablespoons sugar, few gratings lemon rind, and three-fourths tablespoon orange juice. Let simmer until syrup is reduced to two tablespoons, then strain over apple. Chill, and serve with whipped cream.

### Apple Snow.

Wipe, pare, core, and quarter one sour apple. Put in small strainer, place over boiling water, cover, and let steam until apple is soft, then rub through a sieve; there should be one-fourth cup apple pulp. Beat white of one egg until stiff, using a silver fork. Sweeten apple pulp to taste and add gradually to beaten white of egg, continuing the beating. Pile lightly on glass serving-dish, chill, and serve with cream or Steamed Custard.

### Dried Apricot Sauce.

Pick over and wash one-third cup dried apricots, cover with water, and let soak several hours. Cook slowly in same water until soft, adding more water if necessary. Sweeten to taste, and add a few grains salt.

### Strained Apricot Sauce.

Make same as Dried Apricot Sauce, force through a strainer, and add orange juice to taste.

### How to serve a Banana.

Remove skin from a thoroughly ripe banana, and scrape to remove the astringent principle which lies close to skin. Cut in thin slices, arrange on a serving-dish, sprinkle with sugar and a few drops lemon juice.

Banana is served frequently with sugar and cream, but proves difficult of digestion to most people in health; therefore its use would better be avoided for the sick.

### Baked Banana.

Wipe banana and loosen one section of skin, then replace. Put in shallow pan, cover, and bake until skin is very dark, when banana should be soft. Remove from skin, sprinkle with powdered sugar, and serve at once.

### Cranberry Sauce.

Pick over and wash one cup cranberries. Put in saucepan, add one-third cup sugar, and one-third cup water, bring to boiling point, and let boil five minutes. Remove from fire, force through a strainer, and cool.

### Cranberry Jelly.

Pick over and wash one cup cranberries. Put in saucepan, add one-half cup sugar and one-fourth cup water, bring to boiling point and let boil five minutes. Remove from fire, force through a strainer, and pour into individual glass or china moulds. Turn from moulds for serving.

### Stewed Figs.

⅓ cup finely chopped figs.   ½ tablespoon sugar.
¼ cup water.                 1 teaspoon lemon juice.
Few grains salt.

Cook figs, sugar, and water two hours in top of double boiler. Add lemon juice and salt. Chill before serving. One-half tablespoon sherry wine may be added if desired.

### How to serve Grapes.

Put a bunch in colandar and pour over cold water, drain, chill, and arrange on serving-dish. Imperfect grapes, as well as those under ripe or over ripe, should be removed.

A patient should never be allowed to eat grape skins, and in many cases it is desirable to remove grape seeds.

### How to serve Grape Fruit.

Wipe grape fruit and cut in halves crosswise. With a small sharp pointed knife make a cut separating pulp from skin around entire circumference; then make cuts separating pulp from tough portion which divides fruit into sections. Remove tough portion in one piece, which may be accomplished by one cutting with scissors at stem or blossom end close to skin. Sprinkle fruit pulp left in grape fruit skin generously with sugar. Let stand ten minutes, and serve. Place on fruit plate and garnish with a candied cherry.

### Ways of serving Oranges.

1. Wipe orange and cut in halves crosswise. Place one-half on a fruit plate, having an orange spoon or teaspoon on plate at right of fruit.

2. Wipe and cut orange in halves crosswise. Remove pulp and juice, using a spoon. Sprinkle with sugar and serve in a glass dish. Should the orange be allowed to stand for any length of time after the sugar is added, a bitter flavor will be developed.

3. Peel an orange and remove as much of the white portion as possible. Remove pulp by sections, which may be accomplished by using a sharp knife and cutting pulp from tough portion first on one side of section, then on other. Should there be any white portion of skin remaining on pulp it should be cut off. Arrange sections on glass dish or fruit plate. If the orange is a seeded one, remove seeds.

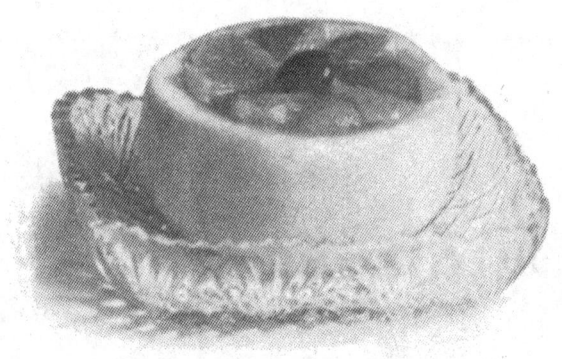

GRAPE FRUIT
See p. 208

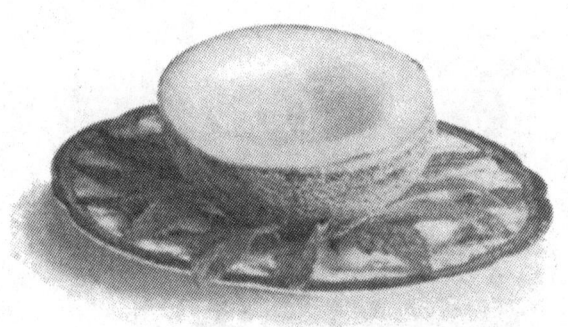

MELON GARNISHED FOR SERVING
See p. 210

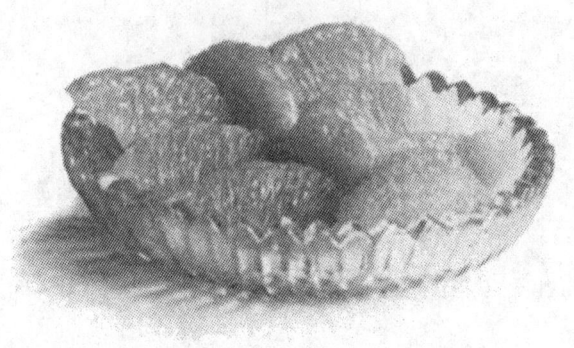

ORANGE PULP
See p. 208

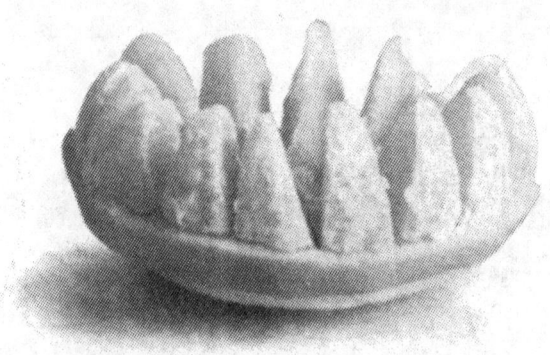

ORANGE PREPARED AND ARRANGED FOR SERVING
See p. 208

FRUITS AND HOW TO SERVE THEM. 209

4. Remove peel from an orange in such a way that there remains a one-half inch band of peel equal distance from stem and blossom end. Cut band, separate sections, and arrange around a mound of sugar.

### Stewed Prunes.

¾ cup prunes.  
1 cup cold water.  
2½ tablespoons sugar.  
Few grains salt.

Wash and pick over prunes. Put in saucepan, add water, and soak two hours; then cook slowly until soft in same water. When nearly cooked add sugar and salt. If soft selected prunes are used, the soaking will not be necessary.

### Baked Pears.

Wipe, quarter, and core pears. Put in earthenware baking-dish, sprinkle with sugar, or add a small quantity of molasses, then add enough water that pears will not burn. Cover, and cook two or three hours in a very slow oven. Seckel pears baked whole are delicious.

### Orange Marmalade.

9 oranges.  
4 lemons.  
8 lbs. sugar.  
4 quarts water.

Wipe fruit and cut crosswise in as thin slices as possible, removing seeds. Put into preserving kettle, cover with the water, and let stand thirty-six hours. Place on range, bring to boiling point, and let boil two hours. Add sugar and let boil one hour. Turn into sterilized jelly tumblers and cover each glass with a circular piece of paraffine paper, then with a larger circular piece of letter paper, fastening paper securely over edge of glass with mucilage.

### Strawberries.

Select one dozen ripe strawberries from which hulls have not been removed. Place in colander, pour over one cup cold water, or, if time allows, dip each one separately in cold water and drain. Arrange around a small mound of powdered sugar. When strawberries are to be served with hulls removed, wash before hulling.

### Peach Snow.

Wipe and remove skin from one peach. Force pulp through a sieve, and if there is much juice, drain. Beat the white of one egg until stiff, using a silver fork. Add peach pulp gradually, while continuing the beating. Sweeten with powdered sugar, pile on glass dish, and serve with Steamed Custard or cream.

### Orange Mint Cup.

Remove pulp from a sour orange. Sprinkle with three-fourths tablespoon powdered sugar, and add one-half tablespoon finely chopped mint, and one teaspoon, each, lemon juice and Sherry. Chill thoroughly. Turn into champagne or frappé glass, and garnish with a sprig of mint.

### How to serve Cantaloup Melon.

Wipe a cantaloup and cut in halves crosswise. Remove seeds and stringy portions. Put one-half melon on fruit plate. Fill with crushed ice and garnish with leaves.

### Fruit Salad I.

Arrange alternate layers of orange pulp, canned shredded pineapple, and sliced banana, sprinkling the layers of orange and banana with powdered sugar. Chill before serving.

### Fruit Salad II.

Arrange alternate layers of orange pulp, strawberries cut in halves lengthwise, and sliced banana, sprinkling each layer with powdered sugar and a few drops lemon juice. Chill, and garnish with whole strawberries and Malaga grapes skinned, seeded, and cut in halves lengthwise.

## CHAPTER XXVIII.

## WAFERS AND CAKES.

### Oat Wafers.

¼ cup rolled oats.
¼ cup wheat preparation.
½ cup flour.
1 tablespoon sugar.
¼ teaspoon salt.
1½ tablespoons butter.
Hot water.

Mix first five ingredients. Work in butter with tips of fingers, and add enough water to hold ingredients together. Toss on a floured cloth, pat, and roll as thinly as possible. Shape with a cutter or cut in strips, using a sharp knife. Bake on a buttered sheet in a slow oven until delicately browned.

These are much enjoyed by a convalescent with a glass of milk or cup of cocoa.

### Scotch Cookies.

1 egg.
¼ cup sugar.
½ cup thick cream.
½ cup fine oatmeal.
2 cups flour.
2 teaspoons baking powder.
1 teaspoon salt.

Beat egg until light, add sugar and cream; then add oatmeal, flour, baking powder, and salt mixed and sifted. Chill mixture. Toss on a floured board, roll, shape with a round cutter, and bake in a moderate oven.

### Wheat Crisps.

⅓ cup butter.
2 tablespoons sugar.
¼ cup milk.
¾ cup wheat preparation.
½ teaspoon salt.
Flour.

Cream the butter, add sugar gradually, milk, wheat preparation mixed with salt, and enough flour to roll.

Roll as thinly as possible, cut in strips four inches long by three-fourths inch wide, and bake in a slow oven.

### Scottish Fancies.

1 egg.
½ cup sugar.
½ tablespoon melted butter.
⅓ teaspoon salt.
¼ teaspoon vanilla.
1 cup rolled oats.

Beat egg until light, add, gradually, sugar, then add remaining ingredients. Drop from tip of spoon on a thoroughly buttered inverted dripping-pan. Spread with a knife, first dipped in cold water, in circular shapes, two inches in diameter. Bake in a slow oven twelve minutes.

### Hot Water Gingerbread.

2 tablespoons molasses.
1 tablespoon boiling water.
4½ tablespoons flour.
⅛ teaspoon soda.
⅛ teaspoon ginger.
Few grains salt.
1½ teaspoons melted butter

Add water to molasses. Mix, and sift dry ingredients; combine mixtures, add butter, and beat vigorously. Bake in individual tins, in a moderate oven fifteen minutes.

### Angel Drop Cakes.

Whites 2 eggs.
¼ teaspoon cream of tartar.
¼ cup fine granulated sugar.
¼ cup flour (sifted four times).
Few grains salt.
⅛ teaspoon vanilla.

Beat whites of eggs until frothy, add cream of tartar, and beat until stiff; then add sugar gradually, while beating constantly, and flavoring. Cut and fold in flour mixed with salt. Drop from tip of teaspoon, one inch apart, on an inverted pan covered with unbuttered paper. Sprinkle with sugar, and bake ten to twelve minutes in a moderate oven.

### Lady Fingers.

Whites 3 eggs.
⅓ cup powdered sugar.
¼ teaspoon vanilla.
Yolks 2 eggs.
⅓ cup flour.
⅛ teaspoon salt.

Beat whites of eggs until stiff and dry, and add sugar gradually, while beating constantly. Beat yolks of eggs until thick and lemon colored. Combine mixtures, add flavoring, then cut and fold in flour mixed and sifted with salt. Shape, using a pastry bag and tube four and one-half inches long and one inch wide on a tin sheet covered with unbuttered paper. Sprinkle with powdered sugar, and bake eight to ten minutes in a moderate oven.

### Sponge Baskets.

| | |
|---|---|
| Yolk 1 egg. | White 1 egg. |
| ⅓ cup sugar. | ⅝ cup flour. |
| 3 tablespoons hot milk or water. | ¾ teaspoon baking powder. |
| ⅛ teaspoon lemon extract. | ⅛ teaspoon salt. |

Beat yolk of egg until thick and lemon colored, add, gradually, one-half the sugar, while beating constantly; then add water or milk, remaining sugar, lemon extract, white of egg beaten stiff, and flour mixed and sifted with salt and baking powder. Bake in buttered gem pans fifteen or twenty minutes. Remove from pan, cool slightly, scoop out centres, and fill with Hamburg cream or whipped cream sweetened and flavored. Insert strips of angelica to represent handles.

### Little Sponge Cakes.

| | |
|---|---|
| Yolks 2 eggs. | Flour. |
| ½ cup sugar. | ¾ teaspoon baking powder. |
| 1⅞ tablespoons cold water. | ⅛ teaspoon salt. |
| ¾ tablespoon corn starch. | Whites 2 eggs |
| ½ teaspoon lemon extract. | |

Beat yolks of eggs until thick and lemon colored, add sugar gradually, and beat two minutes; then add water. Put corn starch in cup and add flour to one-half fill cup. Mix and sift corn starch, flour, baking powder, and salt, and add to first mixture. When well mixed add flavoring, and whites of eggs beaten until stiff. Turn mixture into small tin gem pans previously buttered and floured, sprinkle with sugar, and bake in a moderate oven until delicately browned.

### Sponge Cake.

Yolks 3 eggs.
½ cup sugar.
½ tablespoon lemon juice.
Few gratings lemon rind.
Whites 3 eggs.
½ cup flour.
⅛ teaspoon salt.

Beat yolks of eggs until thick and lemon colored, and add sugar, gradually, while beating constantly. Add lemon juice, rind, and whites of eggs beaten until stiff and dry, folding rather than stirring mixture to keep in as much air as possible; then cut and fold in flour mixed and sifted with salt. Bake forty minutes in a small deep cake pan. The cake should begin to rise during the first ten minutes, continue rising, and begin to brown during the second ten minutes; continue browning during the next ten minutes, and in the last ten minutes finish baking and shrink from the pan. The success of a sponge cake depends upon the amount of air beaten into the eggs and the expansion of that air during baking. A slow oven is necessary for the baking of a genuine sponge cake. So-called sponge cake recipes which call for baking powder require a moderate oven.

### Plain Cake.

1½ tablespoons butter.
¼ cup sugar.
½ egg.
2 tablespoons milk.
7 tablespoons flour.
½ teaspoon baking powder.
Few grains salt.

Cream the butter, add sugar, gradually, and egg well beaten. Mix and sift flour, baking powder, and salt, and add to first mixture alternately with milk. Bake in buttered and floured individual tins, in a moderate oven, twenty minutes. This recipe makes three cakes.

### Cream Cakes.

¼ cup butter.
½ cup boiling water.
2 eggs.
½ cup flour.

Put butter and water in saucepan and place on front of range. As soon as boiling point is reached, add flour all at once, and stir vigorously. Remove from range as soon as mixture begins to leave sides of saucepan, and add unbeaten eggs one at a time, beating until thoroughly mixed between the addition of eggs. Drop by spoonfuls on a buttered sheet one and one-half inches apart, shaping with handle of spoon as nearly circular as possible, having mixture slightly piled in centre. Bake twenty-five minutes in hot oven. Cool, split, and fill with Cream Filling or whipped cream sweetened and flavored.

### Cream Filling.

½ cup sugar.
3 tablespoons flour.
Few grains salt.
1 egg.
1 cup scalded milk.
¼ teaspoon lemon extract.

Mix dry ingredients, add egg slightly beaten, and pour on gradually scalded milk. Cook fifteen minutes in double boiler, stirring constantly until thickened, and afterwards occasionally. Cool and flavor.

### Cereal Macaroons.

White 1 egg.
¼ cup fine granulated sugar.
5 tablespoons wheat preparation.
1 teaspoon vanilla.

Beat white of egg until stiff, add gradually the sugar while beating constantly; then add wheat, and continue beating, and vanilla. Drop from tip of spoon on a buttered sheet one and one-half inches apart. Bake twelve to fifteen minutes in a slow oven.

### Marguerites.

¼ cup sugar.
2 tablespoons water.
¼ cup English walnut meat (finely cut).
White ½ egg.

Boil sugar and water without stirring, until syrup will thread when dropped from tip of spoon; then stir until it begins to grain. Add syrup to white of egg beaten until stiff. Add nut meats and spread on saltines. Bake until delicately browned.

### Meringues or Kisses.

Whites 2 eggs.  ½ cup fine granulated sugar.
¼ teaspoon vanilla.

Beat whites of eggs until stiff, add gradually two-thirds of the sugar while beating constantly, and continue beating until mixture will hold its shape; fold in remaining sugar and add flavoring. Shape with a spoon or pastry bag and tube on wet board covered with buttered paper. Bake thirty minutes in a very slow oven. Remove from paper and put together in pairs; or if intending to fill with ice cream or water ice, remove soft part with spoon and place meringues in oven to dry.

# CHAPTER XXIX.

## DIABETES.

DIABETES means grape sugar in the urine on an ordinary diet. In the first stage of the disease starch turns to sugar; in the second, albumen; and in the third, fat.

Diabetes is essentially a dietetic disease quite common and on the increase during the last forty years. No drug or medicinal remedy has yet been found which is a curative, but prescribed diet keeps the disease under control, and unless the case is severe and of long standing sugar may entirely disappear from the urine. It might seem from this statement that diabetic cures have been accomplished, though such is the case only with the rarest exceptions.

When the disease develops in childhood it is usually severe, but little can be done, and the patient lives but a few weeks or months. There is a case reported by Naunyn in his work on Diabetes mellitus, however, which is an exception to this rule. When the disease develops in adults it is less severe, and life may be prolonged and made pleasurable for many years while of a mild type; when it appears in advanced life it is dangerous on account of complications.

The average daily diet of a man weighing one hundred and fifty-four pounds has been estimated to include:

| Grammes. | | Calories. | | Calories. |
|---|---|---|---|---|
| 500 | × | 4.1 | = | 2050 |
| 125 | × | 4.1 | = | 512.5 |
| 50 | × | 9.3 | = | 465 |
| | | | | 3027.5 |

It may be seen from the above table that the chief source of heat and energy comes from carbohydrates, and it is this class of food that yields the most of the sugar in the body, a small part only being obtained from the proteids.

It is therefore necessary to eliminate the carbohydrates as far as possible, to keep the proteids constant in quantity, or in extreme cases to diminish them and greatly to increase the fats in dietetic diet, allowing two hundred grammes more fat than the daily dietary of a healthy person requires. The change in diet must be a gradual one, as a too sudden reduction of the carbohydrates might prove fatal. Acids are constantly being formed from proteids taken into the body, and these burn in a carbohydrate fire, and acid formation increases when carbohydrates are cut down. The amount further increased, by restricting vegetables, the salts which neutralize these acids are diminished, and if not kept under control will cause acid poisoning. It is an imperative need that there be a movement of the bowels every day. If there be a neglect in this direction patients are more liable to succumb to acid poisoning. Bicarbonate of soda is used in large quantities to aid in the neutralization of the acids.

The first duty of the physician is to decrease the quantity of sugar in the urine, and as far as possible restore the power to assimilate carbohydrates, which is accomplished by resting those functions of the body which are used in the digestion of the same. If the latter is not accomplished the power to assimilate such foods gradually diminishes.

### Proteids in Diet.

The proteids in the diet of the diabetic must be obtained from animal foods, from which he can choose almost without restriction. Meats, fish, and eggs may be indulged in freely. Four to six eggs may be taken daily. Clams, oysters, and mussels contain glycogen (animal starch), which is a carbohydrate, therefore they must be avoided, except in mild forms of the disease, or allowed in restricted amounts. Liver contains so little glycogen that it is practically never necessary to restrict its use.

### Fats in Diet.

Many people have a great repugnance to the use of much fat, therefore the problem of supplying a sufficient quantity to the diabetic is a perplexing one. It must be so combined with other foods as to disguise it as far as possible, and thus avoid the impression on the patient that he is eating a large quantity of fat.

The best fats are butter, cream, eggs, cheese, olive oil, and the fat from bacon, meat, marrow-bone, and oily fish. A diabetic should take at least one-fourth pound butter per day, and one-half pint cream. There is but little tendency to gastric disorders among diabetics, which proves of much assistance in arranging menus.

Green vegetables prove the most efficient butter carriers, spinach heading the list: Other examples, cabbage, asparagus, string beans, etc. If a small quantity of potato is allowable it may take up one-half its weight in butter and one-fourth its weight in heavy cream.

Cream is preferable to milk, and should be used as a substitute for it as far as possible. There is about five per cent of lactose in milk, but only three to four per cent of lactose in cream.

Cheese and olive oil form a very important article in the dietary and may be introduced without much difficulty. From the casein in cheese however sugar is readily formed.

### Vegetables allowed on all Strict Diets.

- Artichokes (French).
- Asparagus.
- Brussels Sprouts.
- Cabbage (red & white).
- Cauliflower.
- Celery-tops.
- Cranberries.
- Cucumbers.
- Horseradish.
- Lettuce.
- Mushrooms.
- Olives.

Onions.
Parsley.
Radishes.
Rhubarb.
Spinach.
String Beans.
Tomatoes.
Water-Cress.

### Fruits allowed.

Only in measured quantities. They contain about ten per cent sugar.

Apples (sour).
Apricots.
Blackberries.
Currants.
Gooseberries.
Grape Fruit.
Lemons.
Oranges.
Peaches.
Plums.
Raspberries.
Strawberries.

Grape fruit and oranges are exceedingly popular and seem especially to agree with diabetics. There is rarely a stage of the disease when an orange or grape fruit cannot be taken once a day.

### Condiments.

The use of condiments is not restricted. Salt, spices, flavoring extracts, vinegar, and table sauces may be used as desired, and are of much help in preparing menus.

### Alcohol.

Brandy, whiskey, rum, gin, claret wine, sour cider, and Bollinger dry champagne are all used, the preference generally being shown for brandy; three to six teaspoons are taken daily, while eight may be allowed. Brandy assists in the digestion of fats. While brandy is constipating under ordinary conditions, it does not prove so with the diabetic on account of the large quantity of fat in his diet.

### Beverages.

One of the symptoms of diabetes is great thirst. Water may be drunk freely; also tea, coffee, and cocoa nibs, without sugar.

## Diabetic Breads.

The most difficult of all starchy foods to take from the diet is ordinary white bread. Many diabetic flours have been placed upon the market which have proved unsatisfactory. Bread made from these flours is seldom liked, and if it is tolerated and eaten in considerable quantity, as large a quantity of starch is taken as when wheat bread containing 55% is used sparingly. A small amount of carbohydrates, especially oatmeal and potato, may be introduced into the dietary on the advice of a physician.

### Standard Diet.

| | Nitrogen. | Carbohydrates. | Fats. | Calories. |
|---|---|---|---|---|
| | Grms. | Grms. | Grms. | $106 \times 4 = 424$ |
| 4 eggs | 4 | | 20 | $55 \times 4 = 220$ |
| 3 oz. cheese | 4 | | 30 | $180 \times 9 = 1620$ |
| 8 oz. meat weighed before cooking | 8 | | 15 | $10 \times 7 = 210$ |
| 2½ oz. bread | 1 | 45 | | 2474 |
| 10 oz. vegetables | | 10 | | |
| 4 oz. butter | | | 100 | |
| ½ oz. olive oil | | | 15 | |
| 10 oz. wine | 0 | 00 | 000 | |
| 30 grms. alcohol ± | | | | |
| | 17 | 55 | 180 | |

17 nitrogen $\times$ 6.25 = 106 proteid.

### Sugar Substitutes.

Saccharine, a cold-tar product three hundred times sweeter than cane sugar, is added to foods for the diabetic. It is usually purchased in the form of tablets. Sustoff, also a chemical substitute, is similar to saccharine, and is just being introduced from Germany into our country. Saccharine is introduced to sweeten beverages and desserts. When used in desserts it must be added at the end of cooking, otherwise a bitter taste is developed. Most patients, after a few months of dieting, prefer to get on without saccharine. When added to sour fruits **it is of benefit in making the food less sour rather than** making it taste sweeter; therefore, avoid the use of too large a quantity. Dissolve a one-half grain tablet in one teaspoon luke-warm water and use as needed, adding cautiously. The amount should not exceed 1½ grains daily.

The one who prepares the food for the diabetic should be in close touch with the doctor, and ever ready and willing to carry out his suggestions. The patient had better not be consulted as regards the menus, nor have his attention called to what he is eating.

It is most unfortunate if it is necessary for the invalid to prepare his own meals, as an appetite for the foods he most needs is greatly diminished. A diabetic should be in the open air as much as possible, and if the condition of the patient admits, walking is preferable to riding.

Frequent feeding is desirable for the diabetic, and besides the three meals, several lunches should be introduced.

### Diabetic Dietary for a Patient whose Urine by Dieting has become Sugar Free.

6.30 A. M. (*before rising*). One cup of coffee with egg.

7.30 A. M. *Breakfast*.
   Fruit — peach, plum, orange, or one-half grape fruit.
   Eggs and fish, or eggs and meat.
   One cup of coffee with cream.

10 A. M. *Lunch*.
   Fruit or cream egg-nog or one cup broth with cream.

12.30 P. M. *Dinner*.
   Soup, fish, meat, two vegetables, or one vegetable and salad; dessert.

3.30 P. M. *Lunch*.
   Cheese sandwich or egg-nog.

6 P. M. *Supper*.
   Eggs, sliced cold meat or fish, cheese, and vegetable or salad.

9 P. M. *Lunch*.
   **Williamson's Diabetic Milk.**

A small piece of white bread, diabetic bread, almond cake, or unsweetened cracker is usually served daily at the time which seems to best please the patient. The quantity is determined by the presence or absence of sugar in the urine.

## RECIPES FOR THE DIABETIC.

### Coffee with Egg.

Use recipe for Boiled or Filtered Coffee (see p. 78). Heat cup, break one egg into cup, and beat slightly with silver fork. Add coffee gradually, stirring constantly, almost filling cup. Sweeten with one-fourth to one-half grain saccharine dissolved in one-half teaspoon cold water. The yolk of the egg may be used in place of the whole egg.

### Coffee with Butter.

Heat cup, put in one teaspoon butter, and add boiled or filtered coffee gradually to almost fill cup. Sweeten, if desired, with saccharine.

### Coffee with Cream.

Pour two-thirds cup boiled or filtered coffee over one tablespoon heavy cream.

### Williamson's Diabetic Milk.

To two cups cold water add one-fourth cup heavy cream and few grains salt; cover, put in ice box, and let stand twelve hours. Remove cover, stir thoroughly, let stand five minutes, and skim off top. Put white one egg in glass, stir, using a silver fork, add one-half cup cold water, and as soon as egg is dissolved, add skimmed cream and a few grains salt. Serve at once.

### Lemonade I.

Add two tablespoons lemon juice to two-thirds cup cold water. Sweeten with one-half grain saccharine dissolved in one teaspoon cold water.

### Lemonade II.

To three tablespoons lemon juice add two-thirds cup cold water, one-eighth teaspoon bicarbonate of soda, and one-half grain saccharine dissolved in one teaspoon cold water.

Lemonade II. is often desirable to relieve the nausea which is caused by the excessive use of fat in the diet.

### Egg Lemonade I.

2 tablespoons lemon juice. ½ grain saccharine dissolved in
White 1 egg. 1 teaspoon water.
⅔ cup cold water.

Add lemon juice to white of egg, and as soon as egg is dissolved add remaining ingredients. Strain and serve.

### Egg Lemonade II.

2 tablespoons lemon juice. ½ grain saccharine dissolved in
1 egg. 1 teaspoon water.
⅔ cup cold water.

Add lemon juice to egg, cover, and shake until well mixed; then add water and saccharine. Strain, and pour from a considerable height from one glass to another.

### Orangeade.

Juice 1 large sour orange. ¼ cup finely crushed ice.
Saccharine.

Pour fruit juice over crushed ice. Sweeten with saccharine if desired.

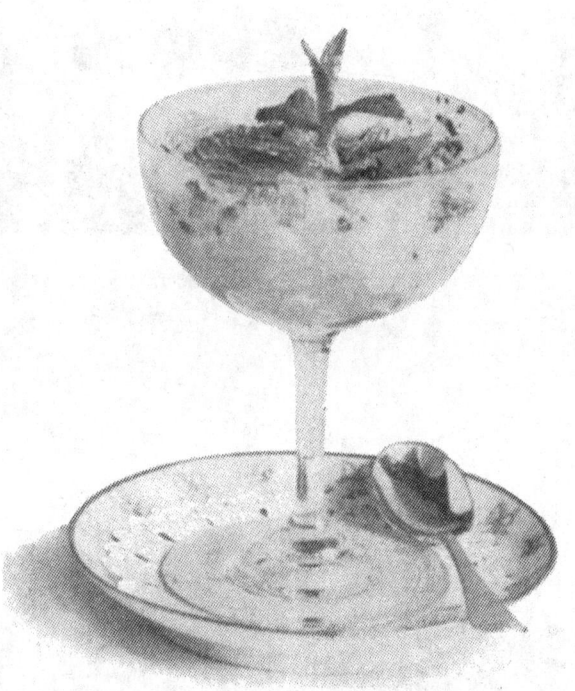

ORANGE MINT CUP
See p. 210

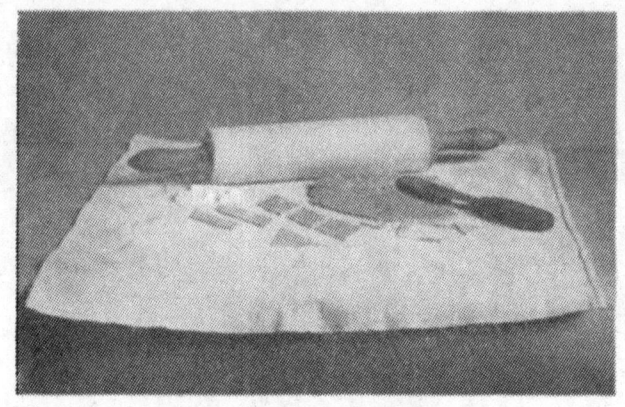

OAT WAFER MIXTURE ILLUSTRATING SHAPING
See p. 211

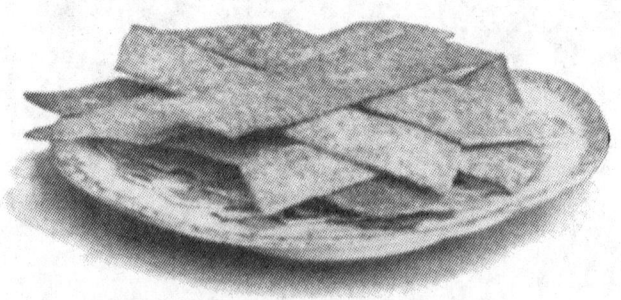

OAT WAFERS
See p. 211

## DIABETES.

### Orange Albumen.

White 1 egg.  
Juice 1 large sour orange.  
¼ cup finely crushed ice.  
Saccharine.

Stir white of egg, using silver fork, and add fruit juice gradually. As soon as egg is dissolved strain over ice. Sweeten with saccharine if desired.

### Claret Albumen.

White 1 egg.  
2 tablespoons claret.  
2 tablespoons finely crushed ice.  
Saccharine.

Beat egg white until stiff, add claret gradually and crushed ice. Sweeten with saccharine if desired.

### Brandy Albumen.

2 teaspoons brandy.  White 1 egg.  
2 tablespoons crushed ice.

Make same as Claret Albumen.

### Cream Egg-Nog.

1 egg.  
1 tablespoon heavy cream.  
¼ cup cold water.  
½ grain saccharine dissolved in 1 teaspoon water.  
Few grains salt.  
Few gratings nutmeg.

Beat egg slightly, add cream diluted with water, dissolved saccharine, salt, and nutmeg. Rum, brandy, or whiskey may be used in combination with nutmeg for flavoring.

### Fruit Egg-Nog.

1 egg.  
2 tablespoons blackberry, raspberry, strawberry, or pineapple juice  
2 tablespoons cold water.  
¼ cup finely crushed ice.  
½ grain saccharine dissolved in 1 teaspoon water.

Mash fresh fruit, put in cheese cloth, and squeeze to express the juice. Beat egg slightly, add water, and gradually fruit juice. Strain, pour over crushed ice, then add saccharine if desired.

### Almond Cakes.

Blanch three-fourths cup almonds, and bake until light brown, then put through almond grater. Place in strainer, and pour over two tablespoons cold water mixed with one tablespoon vinegar; then drain. Dry in oven and grind again. Add four tablespoons melted butter, yolks of five eggs beaten until thick and lemon colored, one-third teaspoon baking powder, and few grains salt. Fold in whites of five eggs beaten until stiff and dry. Fill buttered gem pans two-thirds full, and bake twenty-five minutes in a slow oven. This recipe makes nine cakes.

### Gluten Nut Cakes.

Beat one egg until light, and add one teaspoon melted butter and one-eighth teaspoon salt; then add one-fourth cup almonds (dried in the oven until slightly browned and finely chopped), and one tablespoon Gluten Food. Drop from tip of spoon, and spread in circular shape with back of spoon on a buttered sheet, and cook in a moderate oven until delicately browned.

### Buttered Egg.

Put one teaspoon butter in a small omelet pan. Break one egg into a cup and slip into pan as soon as butter is melted. Sprinkle with salt and pepper and cook until white is firm, turning once during the cooking. Care must be taken not to break the yolk.

### Eggs au Beurre Noir.

Put one teaspoon butter in a small omelet pan. Break one egg into cup, and slip into pan as soon as butter is melted. Sprinkle with salt and pepper and cook until white is firm, turning once during the cooking. Care must be taken not to break the yolk. Remove to hot serving-dish. In same pan melt one-half tablespoon butter and cook until brown, then add one-fourth teaspoon vinegar. Pour over egg.

### Egg à la Suisse.

Heat a small omelet pan and place in it a buttered muffin ring. Put in one-fourth teaspoon butter, and when melted add one tablespoon cream. Break an egg into a cup, slip into muffin ring, and cook until white is set, then remove ring and put cream by teaspoonfuls over egg until the cooking is accomplished. When nearly done sprinkle with salt, pepper, and one-half tablespoon grated cheese. Remove egg to hot serving-dish and pour over cream remaining in pan.

### Dropped Egg with Tomato Purée.

Serve a Dropped Egg (see p. 110) with one tablespoon tomato purée. For tomato purée stew and strain tomatoes, then let simmer until reduced to a thick consistency, and season with salt and pepper and add a few drops vinegar. A grating from horseradish root may be added.

### Egg Farci I.

Cut one " hard boiled " egg in halves crosswise, remove yolk, and rub through a sieve. Clean one-half chicken's liver, finely chop and sauté in just enough butter to prevent burning. While cooking add a few drops onion juice. Add to egg yolk, season with salt, pepper, and one-fourth teaspoon finely chopped parsley. Refill whites with mixture, cover with grated cheese, bake until cheese melts. Serve with one tablespoon tomato purée.

### Egg Farci II.

Prepare egg as for Egg Farci I. Add to yolk one-half tablespoon grated cheese, one-fourth teaspoon vinegar, few grains mustard, and salt and cayenne to taste; then add enough melted butter to make of right consistency to shape. Make into balls size of original yolk and refill whites. Arrange on serving-dish, place in pan of hot water, cover, and let stand until thoroughly heated. Insert a small sprig of parsley in each yolk.

### Baked Egg in Tomato.

Cut a slice from stem end of a medium-sized tomato, and scoop out pulp. Slip an egg into cavity thus made, sprinkle with salt and pepper, replace cover, put in small baking pan, and bake until egg is firm.

### Steamed Egg.

Spread an individual earthen mould generously with butter. Season two tablespoons chopped cooked chicken, veal, or lamb, with one-fourth teaspoon salt and a few grains pepper. Line buttered mould with meat and slip in one egg. Cook in a moderate oven until egg is firm. Turn from mould and garnish with parsley.

### Chicken Soup with Beef Extract.

½ cup chicken stock.   ½ teaspoon Sauterne.
⅛ teaspoon beef extract.   1½ tablespoons cream.
Salt and pepper.

Heat stock to boiling point and add remaining ingredients.

### Chicken Soup with Egg Custard.

Serve Chicken Soup with Egg Custard.

EGG CUSTARD. Beat yolk one egg slightly, add one-half tablespoon, each, cream and water, and season with salt. Pour into a small buttered tin mould, place in pan of hot water, and bake until firm; cool, remove from mould, and cut in fancy shapes.

### Chicken Soup with Egg Balls I. or II.

Serve Chicken Soup with Egg Balls I. or II.

### Egg Balls I.

Rub yolk one "hard boiled" egg through a sieve, season with salt and pepper, and add enough raw egg yolk to make of right consistency to shape. Form into small balls, and poach in soup.

### Egg Balls II.

Rub one-half yolk of "hard boiled" egg through a sieve, add one-half white of "hard boiled" egg finely chopped. Season with salt and pepper and moisten with yolk of raw egg until of right consistency to shape. Form and poach same as Egg Balls I.

### Chicken Soup with Royal Custard.

Serve Chicken Soup with Royal Custard.

ROYAL CUSTARD. Beat yolk one egg slightly, add two tablespoons chicken stock, season with salt and pepper, turn into a small buttered mould, and bake in a pan of hot water until firm. Cool, remove from mould, and cut in small cubes or fancy shapes.

### Onion Soup.

Cook one-half large onion, thinly sliced, in one tablespoon butter eight minutes. Add three-fourths cup chicken stock, and let simmer twenty minutes. Rub through a sieve, add two tablespoons cream, and yolk one-half egg beaten slightly. Season with salt and pepper.

### Asparagus Soup.

| | |
|---|---|
| 12 stalks asparagus, or | Yolk 1 egg. |
| 1/3 cup canned asparagus tips. | 1 tablespoon heavy cream. |
| 2/3 cup chicken stock. | 1/8 teaspoon salt. |
| 1/4 slice onion. | Few grains pepper. |

Cover asparagus with cold water, bring to boiling point, drain, and add to stock and onion; let simmer eight minutes, rub through sieve, reheat, add cream, egg, and seasonings. Strain and serve.

### Tomato Bisque.

| | |
|---|---|
| 2/3 cup canned tomatoes. | 1/8 teaspoon soda. |
| 1/4 slice onion. | 1/2 tablespoon butter. |
| Bit of bay leaf. | 1/4 teaspoon salt. |
| 2 cloves. | Few grains pepper. |
| 1/4 cup boiling water. | 2 tablespoons heavy cream. |

Cook first five ingredients for eight minutes. Rub through sieve, add soda, butter in small pieces, seasonings, and cream. Serve at once.

### Cauliflower Soup.

| | |
|---|---|
| 1/3 cup cooked cauliflower. | 1 egg yolk. |
| 2/3 cup chicken stock. | 1 tablespoon heavy cream. |
| Small stalk celery. | 2 teaspoons butter. |
| 1/4 slice onion. | Salt and pepper. |

Cook cauliflower, stock, celery, and onion eight minutes. Rub through purée strainer, reheat, add egg yolk slightly beaten, cream, butter, and seasonings.

### Mushroom Soup.

| | |
|---|---|
| 3 mushrooms. | 1 egg yolk. |
| 2/3 cup chicken stock. | 1 tablespoon heavy cream. |
| 1/4 slice onion. | 1 teaspoon Sauterne. |
| 2 teaspoons butter. | Salt and pepper. |

Clean mushrooms, chop, and cook in one teaspoon butter five minutes. Add stock, and let simmer eight minutes. Rub through a purée strainer, add egg yolk slightly beaten, cream, remaining butter, seasonings, and wine.

### Spinach Soup.

1 tablespoon cooked chopped spinach.
⅔ cup chicken stock.
Yolk 1 egg.
1 tablespoon heavy cream.
Salt and pepper.

Cook spinach with stock eight minutes. Rub through a purée strainer, reheat, add egg yolk slightly beaten, cream, and seasonings.

### Broiled Fish, Cucumber Sauce.

Serve a small piece of broiled halibut, salmon, or swordfish with cucumber sauce.

### Cucumber Sauce.

Pare one-half cucumber, grate, and drain. Season with salt, pepper, and vinegar.

### Baked Fillet of Halibut, Hollandaise Sauce.

Wipe a small fillet of halibut and fasten with a skewer. Sprinkle with salt and pepper, place in a pan, cover with buttered paper, and bake twelve minutes. Serve with

HOLLANDAISE SAUCE. Put yolk one egg, one tablespoon butter, and one teaspoon lemon juice in small saucepan. Put saucepan in larger one containing boiling water, and stir mixture constantly with a wooden spoon until butter is melted. Then add one-half tablespoon butter, and as mixture thickens another one-half tablespoon butter; season with salt and cayenne. This sauce is almost thick enough to hold its shape. One-eighth teaspoon beef extract, or one-third teaspoon grated horseradish, added to the first mixture, gives variety to this sauce.

### Baked Halibut with Tomato Sauce.

Wipe a small piece of halibut, and sprinkle with salt and pepper. Put in a buttered pan, cover with a very thin strip of fat salt pork gashed several times, and bake twelve to fifteen minutes. Remove fish to serving-dish, discarding pork. Cook eight minutes one-third cup of tomatoes, one-fourth slice onion, one clove, and a few grains salt and pepper. Remove onion and clove, and rub tomato through a sieve. Add a few grains soda and cook until tomato is reduced to two teaspoons. Pour around fish and garnish with parsley.

### Halibut with Cheese.

Sprinkle a small fillet of halibut with salt and pepper, brush over with melted butter, place in pan, and bake twelve minutes. Remove to serving-dish, and pour over the following sauce:

Heat two tablespoons cream, add one-half egg yolk slightly beaten, and when well mixed add one tablespoon grated cheese. Season with salt and paprika.

### Finnan Haddie à la Delmonico.

Cover a small piece finnan haddie with cold water, place on back of range, and allow water to heat gradually to boiling point, then keep below boiling for twenty minutes. Drain, rinse thoroughly, and separate into flakes; there should be two tablespoons. Reheat over hot water with one "hard boiled" egg thinly sliced in two tablespoons heavy cream. Season with salt and paprika, add one teaspoon butter, and sprinkle with finely chopped parsley.

### Fillet of Haddock, White Wine Sauce.

Remove skin from a small piece of haddock, put in buttered baking-pan, pour over one teaspoon melted butter, one tablespoon white wine, and a few drops each lemon juice and onion juice. Cover and bake. Remove to serving-dish, and to liquor in pan add one tablespoon cream and one-half egg yolk slightly beaten. Season with salt and pepper. Strain over fish, and sprinkle with finely chopped parsley.

### Smelts with Cream Sauce.

Clean two selected smelts, and cut five diagonal gashes on sides of each. Season with salt, pepper, and lemon juice. Cover and let stand ten minutes. Roll in cream, dip in flour, and sauté in butter. Remove to serving-dish, and to fat in pan add two tablespoons cream. Cook three minutes, season with salt, pepper, and a few drops lemon juice. Strain sauce around smelts and sprinkle with finely chopped parsley.

### Smelts à la Maître d'Hôtel.

Prepare smelts same as for Smelts with Cream, and serve with Maître d'Hôtel Butter.

### Salt Codfish with Cream.

Pick salt codfish into flakes; there should be two tablespoons. Cover with luke-warm water, and let stand on back of range until soft. Drain, and add three tablespoons cream; as soon as cream is heated add yolk one small egg slightly beaten.

### Salt Codfish with Cheese.

To Salt Codfish with Cream add one-half tablespoon grated cheese and a few grains paprika.

### Broiled Beefsteak, Sauce Figaro.

Serve a portion of broiled beefsteak with Sauce Figaro.
SAUCE FIGARO. To Hollandaise Sauce add one teaspoon tomato purée. To prepare tomato purée stew

tomatoes, force through a strainer, and cook until reduced to a thick pulp.

### Roast Beef, Horseradish Cream Sauce.

Serve a slice of rare roast beef with Horseradish Cream Sauce.

HORSERADISH CREAM SAUCE. Beat one tablespoon heavy cream until stiff. As cream begins to thicken add gradually three-fourths teaspoon vinegar. Season with salt and pepper, then fold in one-half tablespoon grated horseradish root.

### Fillet of Beef.

Wipe a thick slice cut from the tenderloin. Put in hot frying-pan with three tablespoons butter. Sear on one side, turn and sear other side. Cook eight minutes, turning frequently, taking care that the entire surface is seared, thus preventing the escape of the inner juices.

Remove to hot serving-dish and pour over fat in pan first strained through cheese cloth. Garnish with cooked cauliflower, canned string beans, reheated and seasoned, and sautéd mushroom caps.

### Lamb Chops, Sauce Fineste.

Serve Lamb Chops with Sauce Fineste.

SAUCE FINESTE. Cook one-half tablespoon butter until well browned. Add a few grains, each, mustard and cayenne, one-fourth teaspoon Worcestershire Sauce, a few grains lemon juice, and two tablespoons stewed and strained tomatoes.

### Spinach.

Chop one-fourth cooked spinach drained as dry as possible. Season with salt and pepper, press through a purée strainer, reheat in butter, using as much as the spinach will take up. Arrange on serving-dish and garnish with white of "hard boiled" egg cut in strips and yolk forced through a strainer.

### Brussels Sprouts with Curry Sauce.

Pick over Brussels sprouts, remove wilted leaves, and soak in cold water fifteen minutes. Cook in boiling salted water twenty minutes, or until easily pierced with a skewer. Drain, and pour over one-fourth cup

CURRY SAUCE. Mix one-fourth teaspoon mustard, one-fourth teaspoon salt, and a few grains paprika. Add yolk one egg slightly beaten, one tablespoon olive oil, one and one-half tablespoons vinegar, and a few drops onion juice. Cook over hot water, stirring constantly until mixture thickens. Add one-fourth teaspoon Curry powder, one teaspoon melted butter, and one-eighth teaspoon chopped parsley.

### Cauliflower with Hollandaise Sauce.

Serve boiled cauliflower with Hollandaise Sauce.

HOLLANDAISE SAUCE. Put yolk one egg, one tablespoon butter, one teaspoon lemon juice, and one and one-half tablespoons hot water in small saucepan. Put saucepan in larger one containing boiling water and stir mixture constantly, using a wooden spoon, until butter is melted. Add one-half tablespoon butter, and as mixture thickens add another one-half tablespoon butter. Season with salt and cayenne.

### Fried Cauliflower.

Steam a small cauliflower. Cool, and separate into pieces. Sauté enough for one serve in olive oil until thoroughly heated. Season with salt and pepper, arrange on serving-dish, and pour over one tablespoon melted butter.

### Cauliflower à la Huntington.

Separate hot steamed cauliflower into pieces and pour over sauce made same as sauce for Brussels Sprouts with Curry Sauce.

### Celery with Cheese.

Select small stalks of celery having deep grooves, wash, dry, and cut in two-inch pieces. Fill stalks with Neufchâtel cheese, mashed and seasoned with salt and paprika.

### Mushrooms in Cream.

Clean, peel, and break in pieces six medium-sized mushroom caps. Sauté in one-half tablespoon butter three minutes. Add one and one-half tablespoons cream, and cook until mushrooms are tender. Season with salt, pepper, and a slight grating nutmeg.

### Broiled Mushrooms.

Clean mushrooms, remove stems, and place caps on a buttered broiler. Broil five minutes, having gills nearest flame during the first half of broiling. Arrange on serving-dish, put a small piece of butter in each cap and sprinkle with salt and pepper.

### Suprême of Chicken.

Force breast of uncooked chicken through a meat chopper; there should be one-fourth cup. Add one egg beaten slightly, and one-fourth cup heavy cream. Season with salt and pepper. Turn into slightly buttered mould, set in pan of hot water, and bake until firm.

### Meat Soufflé.

½ tablespoon butter.
⅓ tablespoon flour.
2 tablespoons milk.
¼ teaspoon salt.
Few grains pepper.

2 tablespoons cold cooked meat finely chopped.
½ egg yolk.
½ egg white.

Make sauce of first five ingredients, then add meat and egg yolk well beaten. Fold in egg white, beaten until stiff and dry. Turn into a buttered dish, and bake in a slow oven.

### Sardine Relish.

Melt one tablespoon butter, and add two tablespoons cream. Heat to boiling point, add three sardines freed from skin and bones, and separated in small pieces and one "hard boiled" egg finely chopped. Season with salt and cayenne.

### Diabetic Rarebit.

Beat two eggs slightly and add one-fourth teaspoon salt, few grains cayenne, and two tablespoons, each, cream and water. Cook same as Scrambled Eggs, and just before serving add one-fourth Neufchâtel cheese mashed with a fork.

### Cheese Balls.

Mash one-fourth Neufchâtel cheese, using a fork. Add three-fourths teaspoon cracker dust, and season with salt and cayenne. Shape into small balls, dip in beaten egg diluted with water (allowing one tablespoon water to one-half egg), roll in cracker dust, fry in deep fat, and drain on brown paper.

### Cheese Sandwiches.

Cream one-third tablespoon butter and add one-half tablespoon, each, finely chopped cold boiled ham and cold boiled chicken; then season with salt and paprika. Spread between slices of Gruyère cheese cut as thin as possible.

### Cheese Custard.

Beat one egg slightly, add one-fourth cup cold water, two tablespoons heavy cream, one tablespoon melted butter, one tablespoon grated cheese, and a few grains salt. Turn into an individual mould, set in pan of hot water, and bake until firm.

### Cole Slaw.

Select a small heavy cabbage, remove outside leaves, and cut cabbage in quarters; with a sharp knife slice very thinly. Soak in cold water until crisp; drain, dry between towels, and mix with Cream Salad Dressing.

### Cabbage Salad.

Finely shred one-fourth of a small firm cabbage. Let stand two hours in salted cold water, allowing one tablespoon salt to a pint of water. Cook slowly, thirty minutes, one-fourth cup, each, vinegar and cold water with a bit of bay leaf, one-fourth teaspoon peppercorns, one-eighth teaspoon mustard seed, and three cloves. Strain, and pour over cabbage drained from salted water. Let stand two hours, again drain, and serve with or without Mayonnaise Dressing.

### Cabbage and Celery Salad.

Wash and scrape two small stalks celery, add an equal quantity of finely shredded cabbage, and six walnut meats broken in pieces. Serve with Cream Dressing.

### Cucumber Cup.

Pare a cucumber and cut in quarters crosswise. Remove centre from one piece and fill cup thus made with Sauce Tartare. Serve on a lettuce leaf.

### Cucumber and Leek Salad.

Cut cucumber in small cubes and leeks in very thin slices. Mix, using equal parts, and serve with French Dressing.

### Cucumber and Water-cress Salad.

Cut cucumber in very thin slices, and with a three-tined fork make incisions around edge of each slice. Arrange on a bed of water-cress.

### Egg Salad I.

Cut one "hard boiled" egg in halves crosswise in such a way that tops of halves may be left in points. Remove yolk, mash, moisten with cream, French or Mayonnaise Dressing, shape in balls, refill whites, and serve on lettuce leaves. Garnish with thin slices of radish, and a radish so cut as to represent a tulip.

### Egg Salad II.

Prepare egg same as for Egg Salad I., adding to yolk an equal amount of chopped cooked chicken or veal.

### Egg and Cheese Salad.

Prepare egg same as for Egg Salad I., adding to yolk three-fourths tablespoon grated cheese; season with salt, cayenne, and a few grains mustard; then moisten with vinegar and melted butter. Serve with or without salad dressing.

### Egg and Cucumber Salad.

Cut one "hard boiled" egg in thin slices. Cut as many very thin slices from a chilled peeled cucumber as there are slices of egg. Arrange in the form of a circle (alternating egg and cucumber), having slices overlap each other. Fill in centre with chicory or water-cress. Serve with salad dressing.

### Cheese Salad.

Mash one-sixth of a Neufchâtel cheese and moisten with cream. Shape in forms the size of robin's eggs. Arrange on a lettuce leaf and sprinkle with finely chopped parsley which has been dried. Serve with salad dressing.

### Cheese and Olive Salad.

Mash one-eighth of a cream cheese, and season with salt and cayenne. Add two finely chopped olives, two lettuce leaves finely cut, and a small piece of canned pimento to give color. Press in original shape of cheese and let stand two hours. Cut in slices and serve on lettuce leaves with Mayonnaise Dressing.

### Cheese and Tomato Salad.

Peel and chill one medium-sized tomato, and scoop out a small portion of the pulp. Mix equal quantities of Roquefort and Neufchâtel cheese and mash; then moisten with French Dressing. Fill cavity made in tomato with cheese. Serve on lettuce leaves with or without French Dressing.

### Fish Salad I.

Remove salmon from can, rinse thoroughly with hot water and separate in flakes; there should be one-fourth cup. Mix one-eighth teaspoon salt, a few grains each mustard and paprika, one teaspoon melted butter, one-half tablespoon cream, one tablespoon water, one-half tablespoon vinegar and yolk one egg; cook over hot water until mixture thickens; then add one-fourth teaspoon granulated gelatin soaked in one teaspoon cold water. Add to salmon, mould, chill, and serve with

CUCUMBER SAUCE. Beat one tablespoon heavy cream until stiff. Season with salt and pepper, and add, gradually, one teaspoon vinegar, and one-fourth cucumber pared, chopped, and drained.

### Fish Salad II.

Make same as Fish Salad I., using cold cooked flaked cod, halibut, or haddock in place of salmon. Remove from mould, arrange on lettuce leaf, and serve with

CUCUMBER SAUCE. Pare one-fourth cucumber, chop, drain, and add French Dressing to taste.

### Asparagus Salad.

Drain and rinse four stalks canned asparagus. Cut a ring one-third inch wide from a red pepper. Put asparagus stalks through ring, arrange on lettuce leaves, and pour over French Dressing.

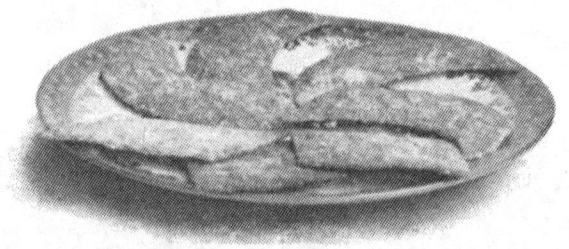

**WHEAT CRISPS**
See p. 211

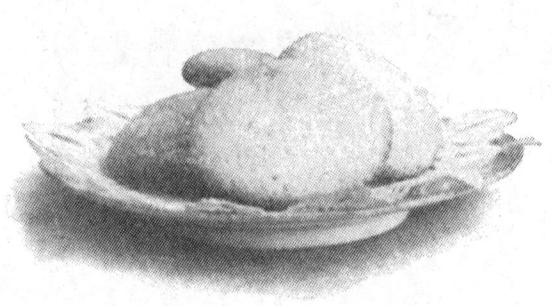

**ANGEL DROP CAKES**
See p. 212

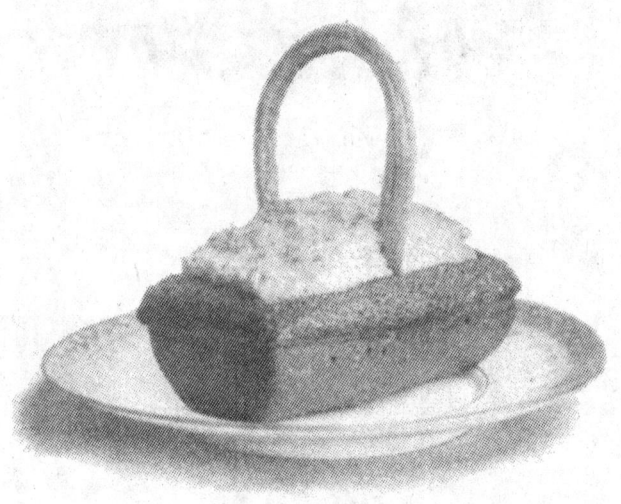

SPONGE BASKET
See p. 213

### Tomato Jelly Salad.

Season one-fourth cup hot stewed and strained tomato with salt, and add one-third teaspoon granulated gelatin soaked in one teaspoon cold water. Turn into an individual mould, chill, turn from mould, arrange on lettuce leaves, and garnish with Mayonnaise Dressing.

### Tomato Jelly Salad with Vegetables.

Cook one-third cup tomatoes with bit of bay leaf, sprig of parsley, one-sixth slice onion, four peppercorns, and one clove, eight minutes. Remove vegetables and rub tomato through a sieve; there should be one-fourth cup. Add one-eighth teaspoon granulated gelatin soaked in one teaspoon cold water, few grains salt, and four drops vinegar. Line an individual mould with cucumber cut in fancy shapes, and string beans, then pour in mixture. Chill, remove from mould, arrange on lettuce leaf, and garnish with Mayonnaise Dressing.

### Frozen Tomato Salad.

Season stewed and strained tomato with salt and cayenne. Fill a small tin box with mixture, cover with buttered paper, then tight fitting cover, pack in salt and ice, using equal parts, and let stand two hours. Remove from mould, place on lettuce leaf, and serve with Mayonnaise Dressing.

### Tomato Basket of Plenty.

Cut a medium-sized tomato in shape of basket, leaving stem end on top of handle. Fill basket with cold cooked string beans cut in small pieces and two halves of English walnut meats broken in pieces, moistened with French Dressing. Serve on lettuce leaves.

### Tomato and Chive Salad.

Remove skin from a small tomato. Chill, and cut in halves crosswise. Spread with Mayonnaise, sprinkle with finely chopped chives, and serve on a lettuce leaf.

### Stuffed Tomato Salad.

Remove skin from a medium-sized tomato and cut slice from stem end. Take out seeds and most of the pulp, and sprinkle inside with salt; invert and let stand one-half hour. Refill with equal parts of finely cut celery and sour apple moistened with Mayonnaise. Serve on shredded lettuce.

### Canary Salad.

Cut a slice from the stem end of a bright red apple, and scoop out pulp, leaving enough to keep shell in shape. Fill shell thus made with grape fruit pulp and finely cut celery, using twice as much grape fruit as celery. It will be necessary to drain some of the juice from the grape fruit. Moisten with Mayonnaise Dressing, replace cover, arrange on lettuce leaf, and garnish with a canary made by mashing Neufchâtel cheese, coloring yellow, and shaping, designating eyes with paprika and putting a few grains on body of bird. Also garnish with three eggs made from cheese colored green and speckled with paprika.

### Harvard Salad.

Cut a selected lemon in the form of a basket with handle, and scoop out all pulp. Fill basket thus made with one tablespoon cold cooked chicken or sweetbread cut in small dice, mixed with one-half tablespoon small cucumber dice and one teaspoon finely cut celery, moistened with cream or Mayonnaise Dressing. Spread top with dressing and sprinkle with thin parings cut from round red radishes finely chopped. Insert a small sprig of parsley in top of handle. Arrange on water-cress.

### Cucumber Boats.

Cut a small cucumber in halves lengthwise. Scoop out centres and cut boat shaped. Cut cucumber removed from boats in small pieces and add one and one-half olives finely chopped. Moisten with French Dressing, fill boats with mixture, and arrange on lettuce leaves.

### Spinach Salad.

Drain and finely chop one-fourth cup cooked spinach. Season with salt, pepper, lemon juice, and melted butter. Pack solidly into an individual mould, chill, remove from mould, and arrange on a thin slice of cold cooked tongue cut in circular shape. Garnish base of mould with a wreath of parsley and top with

SAUCE TARTARE. To one tablespoon Mayonnaise Dressing add three-fourths teaspoon finely chopped capers, pickles, olives, and parsley, having equal parts of each.

### Sweetbread and Cucumber Salad.

Mix two tablepoons cold cooked sweetbread cut in cubes, one tablespoon cucumber cubes, and one-half tablespoon finely cut celery. Beat one and one-half tablespoons heavy cream until stiff, then add one-eighth teaspoon granulated gelatin dissolved in one teaspoon boiling water and three-fourths teaspoon vinegar. Set in pan of ice water, and as mixture begins to thicken add sweetbread and vegetables. Mould and chill. Remove from mould, arrange on lettuce leaves, and garnish top with a slice of cucumber and a sprig of parsley.

### Chicken and Nut Salad.

Mix two tablespoons cold cooked chicken or fowl cut in cubes with one tablespoon finely cut celery and one-half tablespoon English walnut meats browned in oven with one-eighth teaspoon butter and a few grains salt, then broken in pieces. Moisten with Mayonnaise Dressing. Mound and garnish with curled celery, tips of celery, and whole nut meats.

### Apple Velvet Cream.

¼ cup steamed and strained apple
½ saccharine tablet dissolved in
½ teaspoon cold water.
1 teaspoon granulated gelatin dissolved in
2 teaspoons boiling water.
½ egg white beaten stiff.
1½ tablespoons heavy cream beaten stiff.
1 teaspoon lemon juice.
Few grains salt.

Mix ingredients in order given. Turn into a mould and chill.

### Coffee Bavarian Cream.

2 tablespoons coffee infusion.
1 tablespoon water.
2 tablespoons heavy cream.
1 egg yolk.
Few grains salt.
¾ teaspoon granulated gelatin soaked in
1 teaspoon cold water.
1 grain saccharine dissolved in ½ teaspoon cold water.
1 egg white.
¼ teaspoon vanilla.

Scald coffee, water, and one-half cream. Add egg yolk slightly beaten, and cook until mixture thickens; then add gelatin and salt. Remove from fire, cool, add saccharine, remaining cream beaten until stiff, egg white beaten until stiff, and teaspoon vanilla. Turn into a mould and chill.

### Princess Pudding.

1 egg yolk.
¾ teaspoon granulated gelatin dissolved in
1 tablespoon boiling water.
2 teaspoons lemon juice.
¼ grain saccharine dissolved in
¼ teaspoon cold water.
1 egg white.

Beat egg yolk until thick and lemon colored, and add gelatin, continuing the beating. As mixture thickens add gradually lemon juice and saccharine. Fold in white of egg beaten until stiff and dry. Turn into a mould and chill.

## Lemon Cream Sherbet.

¼ cup cream.
2 tablespoons cold water.
½ grain saccharine dissolved in
½ teaspoon cold water.
4 drops lemon juice.
Few grains salt.

Mix ingredients in order given, and freeze.

## Orange Ice.

⅓ cup orange juice.
1 teaspoon lemon juice.
½ grain saccharine dissolved in
½ teaspoon cold water.
2 tablespoons cold water.

Mix ingredients in order given, and freeze.

## Grape Fruit Ice.

¼ cup grape fruit juice.
¼ cup water.
½ grain saccharine dissolved in
½ teaspoon cold water.

Remove juice from grape fruit, strain, add remaining ingredients, and freeze to a mush.

Serve in sections of grape fruit.

## Frozen Punch.

¼ cup cream.
2 tablespoons cold water.
1 ½ teaspoons rum.
Yolk 1 egg.
½ grain saccharine dissolved in
½ teaspoon cold water.
Few grains salt.

Scald one-half cream with water, add egg yolk slightly beaten, and cook over hot water until mixture thickens. Cool, add remaining ingredients, and freeze.

## French Pudding.

⅔ cup cream.
White 1 egg.
Few grains salt.
⅛ teaspoon vanilla.
Sliced fruit.

Heat cream. Beat white of egg until stiff, add salt, vanilla, and cream, and beat with egg-beater. Turn into buttered individual moulds and bake until firm. Serve cold with sliced fruit.

## CHAPTER XXX.

### DIET IN SPECIAL DISEASES.

#### CONSTIPATION.

CONSTIPATION is due, usually, to a neglect in attending to the calls of nature. Those suffering from constipation should never forget the importance of regularity in this matter and should see to it each day at a fixed time. This regularity, without other treatment, often rids one of the complaint.

Physical exercise and regularity in meals also play an important part towards keeping the bowels in a healthy condition. Those of sedentary habits are more liable to constipation than those engaged in a more active out-of-door life.

Oftentimes cases of constipation may be overcome by a suitable diet. If diet alone will not effect a cure, then diet with some medicinal remedy must be tried.

The simplest remedy is the increase of water in the dietary. Cold water taken before breakfast and upon retiring increases peristalsis. Many of the saline waters are used to advantage.

Coarse foods are recommended always for constipation. Such foods contain a large quantity of cellulose, and include cereals, coarse breads, vegetables, and fruits. They are bulky, slightly irritating, and leave much residue in the intestine. There is danger if such foods are taken in excess, as the bowels become tired from over stimulation and fail to react.

Cookery plays a very important part in the digestion of foods. Cereals, coarse breads, and vegetables, if properly and thoroughly cooked, are well digested, and at

## DIET IN SPECIAL DISEASES.

the same time leave a sufficient residue to stimulate the intestines to action.

Fruits, on account of the organic acids present, act as a laxative, and should be used between meals as well as at meals. The juice expressed from two oranges may be taken early in the morning to great advantage. Among the dried fruits, figs, prunes, dates, and raisins, cooked or uncooked, are useful in cases of constipation.

Fats and oils tend to produce a laxative condition. If they have been introduced sparingly in the diet, they may be gradually increased until used in moderation.

The foods most constipating are those that are well digested and most completely absorbed. An egg is an example of this kind of food. Milk seems to furnish an exception to this rule, for although it leaves considerable residue in the intestine it is recognized as a constipating food.

### DIARRHŒA.

Diarrhœa is a frequent evacuation of the bowels. If the case is a mild one, rest and quiet, with a small supply of liquid foods, which yield little residue, will effect a cure. In severe cases it is sometimes necessary to abstain from all food for a short time, giving the entire body, as far as possible, complete rest. A patient quickly loses strength by withholding food, nevertheless it seems the best course to pursue. Hot water may be administered by the teaspoonful, and this may be followed by thin oatmeal gruel or rice water. Albumen water, tea, and blackberry and red wines may be introduced to advantage. Tea, and blackberry and red wines act as an astringent on account of the tannin they contain.

From thin gruels gradually work up to thicker ones, and introduce milk into their preparation with some lime water. Frequently an egg may be added. Thin cream is well borne in teaspoonful doses.

Scraped raw or rare roast beef and crackers may be added to the dietary as the condition of the patient improves. Preparations containing meat extracts always should be avoided, as well as aerated water, and, above all, cold milk, which would prove disastrous.

## STOMACH TROUBLES.

The secret of good digestion lies largely in the proper cooking and mastication of foods which have been wisely selected. Regular hours for meals should also be observed if one wishes to avoid stomach troubles.

The causes of stomach trouble, commonly called indigestion, are so many as to be almost without number. Over-feeding, under-feeding, improper feeding, late suppers, poor ventilation, overwork, want of exercise, worry, nervous anxiety, depression of spirits, all tend to retard the work of the digestive system. It seems to be the office of the physician to locate the cause and try as far as possible to alleviate the suffering by making changes in diet and administering medicine.

Indigestion is usually located in the stomach, causing faintness, fullness, flatulency, hyper-acidity, or dilation. Sick headaches too are frequently caused by indigestion.

Patients afflicted with chronic gastric troubles are more apt to under-eat than over-eat. When one is suffering from malnutrition as well as stomach trouble, the system is so reduced that the body as a whole needs to be considered as well as the stomach. In dealing with such patients their personal idiosyncrasies must be considered. Perhaps there is no disease in which they play a more important part.

Rest after meals is always to be recommended, which is best accomplished by lying down for fifteen minutes or even longer.

## HYPER-ACIDITY OF THE STOMACH.

One of the commonest forms in which indigestion appears is hyper-acidity of the stomach, which is due to an excessive amount of gastric juice. This condition greatly delays the passing on of the food into the duodenum by retarding the opening of the pylorus.

A delay of food in the stomach favors the development of bacteria, also causing acid fermentation. It is wise to restrict albuminous food by cutting down the quantity of meat. A diet composed largely of meat produces an excess of acid in the gastric juice.

Introduce milk into the dietary, which, being without extractives, calls forth the least gastric juice of all proteid food. Eggs are likewise desirable. It is well to increase the fat in the form of butter, cream, and olive oil. Begin by taking one-fourth cup of cream daily, and make a gradual increase until one-half cup is consumed. Fats seem to restrain the flow of gastric juice even in the presence of other foods. The amounts of carbohydrate food may be slightly increased, and some of the various malt preparations may be used to advantage. Hot water, as well as diluting the contents of the stomach, increases the frequency and the vigor of its muscular movements, therefore its use is advised. Warmth always tends to stimulate the opening of the pyloric. Where expense is not considered alkaline waters taken with meals prove beneficial.

Restrict the use of foods that increase the acidity of the urine, namely, — spinach, rhubarb, water-cress, sorrel, tea, coffee, etc. Foods containing oxalic acid under ordinary conditions produce no harmful results, as so large an amount of the acid is unabsorbed, while if hyper-acidity of the stomach is present this acid is so well absorbed that it leads to trouble.

It is a common practice to take magnesia to neutralize an acid condition of the stomach, but such a treatment is not to be recommended.

## ULCER OF THE STOMACH.

Ulcer of the stomach requires rest and restriction of all food by the mouth.

A nutritive enema should be given every six hours, six ounces being administered each time, consisting of one raw egg, one-fourth teaspoon salt, and one-half cup milk. When this quantity is found to be well retained, gradually increase the quantity one ounce at a time until nine ounces are consumed. One teaspoon sugar may be added to each enema.

An enema of water at body temperature should be given once during every twenty-four hours for the purpose of washing out the bowels, which greatly assists in the absorption of rectal feeding. An occasional enema of salt solution may be given, allowing one teaspoon salt to one pint water.

When pain and vomiting have ceased, nourishment may be taken by the mouth, beginning with a thin water-oatmeal gruel, administering two teaspoons every two hours, and gradually increasing the amount to the limit of from one-half to three-fourths of a cup. If the water-gruel is well borne, introduce milk into its preparation, followed by milk to which lime water is added. Cocoa, chicken broth with rice, crackers, softened toast, and rennet may next be used. Never allow soups rich in extractives, and even in advanced convalescence avoid the use of irritating or indigestible forms of food.

## GASTRITIS.

The feeding in gastritis should be along the same lines as for ulcer of the stomach, rectal feeding seldom being necessary.

While all food should be withheld as long as the patient continues to vomit, to relieve thirst occasional sips of hot water may be allowed or small pieces of crushed ice may be held in the mouth. If the case is chronic, any food that will irritate the gastric mucous membrane or excite a secretion of mucus must be avoided.

Spices and condiments are forbidden, alcohol is prohibited, and usually coffee on account of the oil which it contains; weak tea, however, is allowed. Cane sugar causes an outpouring of a large quantity of mucus in the stomach, which greatly retards the digestion of other foods; consequently, if taken at all, must be used in very small quantities. Dextrose and lactose are much less liable to be harmful.

Fat in the form of butter is well borne; cooked fat of meats, sauces, and pastries would better be avoided.

Bread should be thoroughly toasted, that the starch may be dextrinized. Such vegetables as contain a small quantity of cellulose may be used, and they should be served in a finely divided state. Potato purée, chopped spinach, and cauliflower furnish excellent illustrations of vegetables to be served to the sufferer of gastritis.

## DILATED STOMACH.

Dilation of the stomach may be the result of a run-down condition of the system, when for some reason the walls of the stomach have become weakened, or the opening from the stomach to the duodenum has become small. Whatever the cause, the result is the same, namely, the food remains in the stomach longer than it ought, giving rise to acetic, butyric, and lactic fermentation, and $CO_2$ gas is liberated. The large quantity of fermented food causes an excess of gastric juice.

A striking example of a dilated stomach has been furnished by a woman who lost her right arm, and who obtained her livelihood by keeping a small store, from which fact her meals were often interrupted by customers; consequently her food was poorly divided as well as improperly masticated.

If the case is not a severe one, great relief may be obtained by taking thoroughly cooked food that will not ferment in small quantities, and finely dividing and masticating the same. Beside the three meals, three luncheons should be introduced each day. The use of water must be restricted.

An hour's rest in a reclining position is necessary after each meal, and the patient should be so raised as to assist the food in its passage from the stomach.

The temperature of foods must be considered in feeding the patient. All cold foods cause distress.

In the treatment of all stomach troubles, it is necessary to consider the quantity of gastric juices poured out. Albumen, as found in eggs and milk, calls forth very little gastric juice, while fats call forth none.

The washing out of the stomach once each day in severe cases seems imperative; and this treatment needs to be followed for several months, or until such time as there is no appearance of undigested food in the withdrawn contents

In restricting the amount of water in the dietary, it may be necessary to inject salt and water by the rectum. If the patient suffers no especial inconvenience, the amount of urine passed may drop from three pints, the usual daily amount, to one pint.

**Suggestions as to the Menu for a Patient suffering from a Dilated Stomach.**

*Breakfast:*
 Strained cereal.
 Cream.
 1 slice buttered toasted bread.
 1 egg.
 Coffee.
 2 lumps sugar.

A. M. *Luncheon:*
 Glass of milk.
 Stale bread, rusk or cracker.

*Dinner:*
  Roast beef or beefsteak.
  Vegetable (that may be finely divided).
Example : Mashed potato, finely chopped spinach, asparagus tips, etc.
  These vegetables will take up quite a little butter.
  Simple Dessert, as Junket, custard, etc.
P. M. *Luncheon:*
  Glass of milk with a cracker or
  Raw egg.
*Supper:*
  Creamed Toast.
  Cold meat (thinly sliced).
*Before retiring:*
  Glass of milk.
  Cracker.

## HOW TO INCREASE BODY WEIGHT.

A fattening diet is called for under the following conditions : —
1. To store up fat.
2. During convalescence after acute disease.
3. In chronic wasting diseases.
4. In some nervous diseases.

There are many persons in apparent health who need to store up fat in order that they may be better fortified against disease, and that they may look better, not giving the appearance of malnutrition. In order to accomplish this, rest and diet must be considered.

When thin people have exercised freely, cut down the exercise as far as is practicable to increase body weight. The three meals must be given regularly and luncheons introduced. A weekly gain of one pound is better than a more rapid increase.

Experience has proved that milk is an excellent kind of food to use in the diet. Begin by taking two tablespoons at the close of each meal and between meals. The amount to be increased by the addition of one tablespoon at each daily serving until a glassful is consumed. Milk, when taken for luncheons, should be served with a small cracker. Milk should always be sipped rather than drunk, and fifteen minutes should be employed in taking a glassful.

Fats in an easily digested form burn slowly, have the advantage of much nutriment in small bulk, and are easily stored in the system as fats. For these reasons they are highly recommended for the fattening process, though they must be considered as expensive forms of food. There is danger, however, if they are used to excess, of overtaxing the digestion; therefore carbohydrates as well as fats must be well represented in the diet.

In general, carbohydrates are sufficiently used in the diet from the fact that most people have a natural craving for sweets; then again, both sugars and starches are inexpensive forms of food.

Cream is a most acceptable form of fat, and is well borne and liked by most people. Like milk, it is well to introduce it gradually into the dietary, never allowing the quantity to exceed one-half cup daily. Encourage a free use of butter, as it holds high place both as regards digestibility and as a fattening agent. Vegetables are the best known butter carriers.

A salad served with an oil dressing should be found in the daily dietary. If olive oil does not prove an agreeable addition to salads, the oil may be taken by spoonful doses at the close of each meal to advantage, and even though not enjoyed may be tolerated and endured.

Among the fats of meats, bacon fat is especially well liked. The fats of other meats have been probably sparingly eaten or ignored in the dietary of a thin person.

It is always wise to consider the tastes of the patient as far as possible in introducing an excess of fat into the dietary. If an occasional change is made, less emphasis is laid upon its use.

DIET IN SPECIAL DISEASES. 255

One, two, or three eggs may be introduced daily as liked. The yolks of eggs contain a considerable quantity of fat, and it must never be forgotten that eggs are a valuable proteid food.

Fruits stimulate the appetite and are often acceptable when served with cream. Alcoholic stimulants should not be used; while beer and malt liquors are fattening their use would better be avoided except under the doctor's order.

## OBESITY.

An excess of fat is almost invariably due to too much food with too little exercise. There are exceptional cases of obesity where only a moderate supply of food causes an excess of fat, but they are of less frequency than is usually supposed. Over-indulgence in diet is not uncommon to those of large incomes, and obesity usually follows, especially where little exercise is taken. It seems easy for such victims to deceive themselves as to the real cause of their complaint and attribute it to inherited tendencies. They generally assert "it belongs to our family to be fat." Although some truth lies in this statement, a restricted diet, with sufficient exercise, must exert a change in the right direction.

To treat obesity there must be a reduction in the amount of food or an increase in the amount of work, and sometimes both these considerations need play a part. It has been found safer to cut down the number of calories given rather than to restrict the use of any especial class of foods.

A patient is quite likely to suffer from weakness and faintness when there is a loss of flesh occasioned by the cutting down of the food supply. These symptoms are overcome partially if, besides the three meals, three luncheons are introduced.

In reducing the food supply, see to it that the proteids (tissue building foods) are in sufficient quantity to keep up the strength of the patient. Van Noorden asserts that one hundred and fifty-five grammes of albumen should be taken daily.

It is desirable to cut off the fat in meats and avoid all kinds of fat meat and restrict the use of milk, except the small quantity that may be used with tea or coffee. Buttermilk, if liked, is a desirable beverage.

Both sugars and starches should be used sparingly; therefore the supply of bread, potatoes, and cereals during periods of diet should be cut down to a very limited supply, while sweet desserts would better be avoided.

Fruits and vegetables, being bulky foods, are well used with meats and eggs, which are concentrated foods.

Water, saline waters, tea, and coffee are allowed as beverages if taken in moderation. Alcohol should be avoided, but in cases of weak heart-action it is sometimes necessary to resort to its use; then whiskey may be taken in teaspoon doses; also some wines containing a small percentage of sugar. Strong, sweet wines, liqueurs, and malt liquors should not be allowed.

After all is said and done, experience has shown that no stated rules can be laid down for the treatment of the over-fat. Individual cases call for individual diets. In some it seems well to cut down the fats more than any other class of foods; in others, the carbohydrates. It is a safe statement to make that the number of calories should be decreased about one-fifth from the standard to bring about the best results, which is a loss of body weight of about one-half pound weekly. In extreme cases the calories are cut two-fifths with satisfying results, but with greater loss of body weights. When such a diet is resorted to it would better be adhered to for about one month, then a return made to a normal diet, followed by another period of restricted diet.

When obesity is accompanied by heart trouble, then the greatest care must be taken as regards the food supply, and the patient's symptoms must be carefully watched.

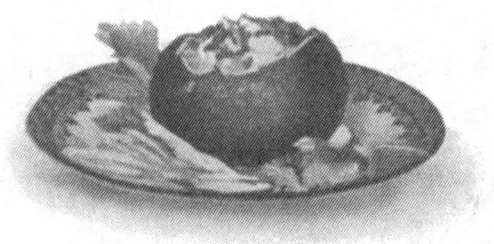

STUFFED TOMATO SALAD
See p. 242

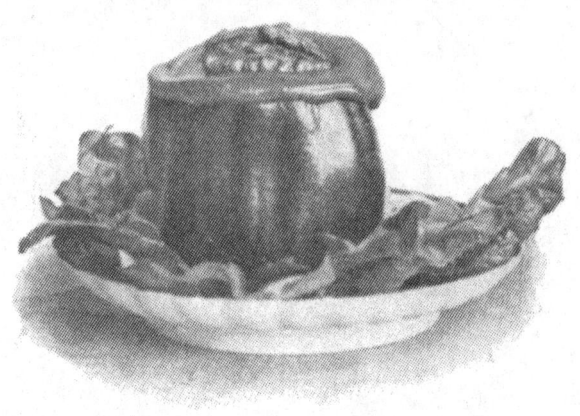

CELERY AND GRAPE FRUIT SALAD SERVED IN
GREEN PEPPER

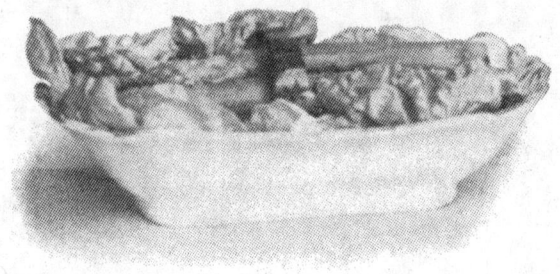

**ASPARAGUS SALAD**
See p. 240

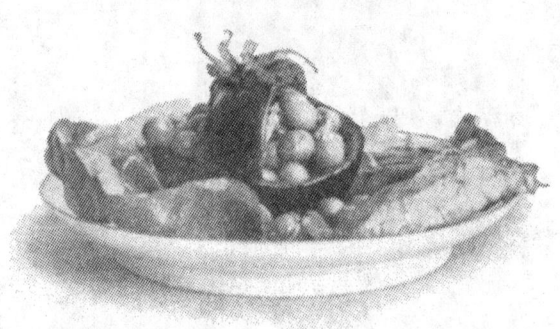

**TOMATO BASKET, WITH PEAS**
See p. 241

## TYPHOID FEVER.

Typhoid fever is a germ disease, infectious while not contagious, located in the small intestines. It is not possible to contract typhoid by contact with the patient, but danger lies from contact with the fæces; therefore too much stress cannot be laid upon the immediate disinfection and disposal of the same.

Typhoid is largely attributable to an impure milk or water supply, while cases are recorded from the eating of raw oysters which have been contaminated from sewage which contained typhoid bacilli.

If a physician were asked off-hand what he would recommend for the feeding of a typhoid patient, he would say, most likely, feed the patient to the limit of his digestive capacity, which may be determined by the condition of his stools.

No amount of food given to a fever patient is capable of establishing nitrogenous equilibrium, as there is such a rapid destruction of nitrogenous tissues. The microorganisms which produce typhoid have a marked destroying influence on the proteid constituents of the body. From this statement one might draw the deduction that a large supply of proteid food should be furnished, but this would add to the waste products, which are already excessive, thus overtaxing the kidneys, which would be harmful rather than beneficial. Tissue-sparing foods may be liberally supplied in the diet in a carbohydrate form, as fats usually prove repugnant to a fever patient. Gelatin, although classed under proteids, is valuable, principally, as a proteid sparer, although its final products are similar to the final products of all proteids.

During the last few years an exclusive milk diet has been used by many physicians and in almost all hospitals, but the best authorities are now agreed that while milk should furnish the principal article of diet, other foods may be introduced advantageously, namely: Koumiss, junket, orange albumen, strained oatmeal and wheat gruels, chicken and mutton broth, soft-cooked eggs, bread, jellies, ice cream, and in some cases a small piece of broiled beefsteak or breast of chicken is allowed.

Typhoid patients always require frequent feedings, — usually every two hours during the day and several times during the night. There is a craving for cold water, which may be gratified, but it is best to restrict the quantity at any one time. Fruit beverages may be indulged in freely, as much water is ingested by their use. They are often fortified by the use of lactose for sweetening. Lactose has advantages over cane sugar, as it is less sweet to the taste, and under ordinary conditions does not ferment.

When a strictly milk diet is depended upon, there is great danger of under-feeding the patient. The amount should never fall below three pints daily, and two quarts is usually considered necessary. When milk is diluted with alkaline or effervescent waters, to make it more palatable or more easily digested, it must be remembered that its nutritive value is greatly diminished, a fact often overlooked by those caring for the sick. Koumiss is a form of milk which is well borne by typhoid patients.

To make a liquid or semi-liquid diet bearable for any length of time without destroying all desire for food, it is necessary to offer as much variety as possible, and for this reason chicken and mutton broth are given to stimulate appetite rather than for their food value. Beef tea should never be allowed, as the extractives of beef are liable to excite diarrhœa, which, above all symptoms, is to be avoided.

## RHEUMATISM.

In the dietetic treatment of rheumatism physicians differ greatly, but on one point they seem agreed, namely: That a moderate diet of well-cooked simple food must be enforced. Much out-of-door life is strongly

DIET IN SPECIAL DISEASES. 259

recommended, with moderate exercise, and cold-water baths are usually found to be beneficial.

Foods rich in extractives are avoided, also tea, coffee, and alcohol in all its forms. Beef is considered more stimulating than lamb or chicken, and is excluded from the dietary. Sweetbreads give rise to uric acid in the system, therefore they must be condemned by the sufferer from rheumatism.

Cereals, milk, eggs, fresh fruit, and vegetables should form the principal part of the diet, and above all, good eating habits should be established, which consist of regularity of meals as well as a sufficient time for eating the same. Late suppers always should be avoided.

## BRIGHT'S DISEASE.

Bright's disease is a disease of the kidneys, and is recognized by the persistent presence of albumen in the urine, and the wasting of the affected organ. Bright's disease may be acute or chronic, and in either case rest the organ as far as possible. This may be accomplished by avoiding work or irritants for the kidney. The physician recognizes the fact that the kidney is but a small part of the body, therefore does not forget to consider the body as a whole, and especially the heart, as that organ is overtaxed.

In acute cases of Bright's disease the use of water is restricted to a moderate supply, one pint to two quarts daily. Formerly, in chronic cases, water was given freely, with the thought that thereby waste products might be more readily excreted. Van Noorden claims that waste products are excreted quite as well in a small as in a large quantity of urine, and his theory is verified by other noted authorities.

A milk diet, in extreme cases, was formerly considered a safe one to follow. At the present time it is looked upon with suspicion, and the amount given should not exceed a quart. Van Noorden asserts that too much albumen is given if more than that quantity is allowed, a theory now adopted by the leading physicians of our own country.

Albumen, in acute cases, for a time must be restricted, but as the disease becomes chronic care must be taken that the supply is sufficient for the needs of the body. It should not exceed forty-five grammes, however. From whatever source albumen is supplied its effect upon the urine is identical.

While it has not been proved that meats are distinctly harmful, the quantity in the diet is of necessity restricted, on account of the albumen they contain.

White meats are preferable to red meats, only because a smaller quantity is usually desired.

Eggs, vegetables free from albumen (e. g. potatoes, rice), and fruits, being deficient in extractives, furnish desirable foods for the sufferer from Bright's disease. Fats may also be given. In chronic cases the amount of albumen given daily should not fall below forty-five grammes, and as a rule a larger amount is furnished.

Among condiments salt may be used only very sparingly, since the kidneys do not excrete it well.

### Foods and Condiments not allowed.

| | |
|---|---|
| Alcoholic Stimulants. | Garlic. |
| Anise. | Leeks. |
| Asparagus. | Mushrooms. |
| Caraway. | Mustard. |
| Cayenne. | Paprika. |
| Celery | Pepper. |
| Clove. | Sorrel. |
| Coffee. | Tea. |
| Curry Powder. | Truffles. |

Vinegar, being oxidized in the body, is allowed, and there seems to be no reason why lemon juice may not be

DIET IN SPECIAL DISEASES. 261

taken, although it has been thought harmful by many. Alcohol in any form should be avoided. Exception must be made to Kefir and Koumiss, which are allowed in moderation, as they contain so small a quantity. Tea and coffee are forbidden on account of their action on the heart. The use of tobacco is avoided for the same reason.

Apart from the dietary, a warm climate, with hot baths, frequent bowel movements, and a reclining position assist materially in the treatment of the disease.

### A Day's Ration in Acute Case.

| | | | | | |
|---|---|---|---|---|---|
| Milk . . . | 1000 | grammes | . . . | 600–700 | calories. |
| Cream . . | 250 | " | . . . | 600–700 | " |
| Rice . . . | 50 | " | (or more) | 175 | " |
| Toast . . | 50 } | | | | |
| or | } | " | (or more) | 125 | " |
| Potato . . | 125 } | | | | |
| Fresh Butter | 30 | " | (or more) | 250 | " |
| | | | | 1750 calories. | |

## CONSUMPTION (PHTHISIS).

It is frequently the case that the illy nourished fall victims to phthisis, and the danger is increased if one has inherited tendencies to the disease. Statistics show that the death rate from phthisis is alarmingly large, and it might be materially lessened, and in a few years eradicated, if the strictest attention was paid to the burning of all sputum.

On account of the great destruction of tissues in the consumptive, there should be given a generous supply of tissue-forming foods. The rations should be of such a character that they may be easily digested, and they should be given at regular, frequent intervals. Besides breakfast, dinner, and supper, there should be a luncheon in the morning, another in the afternoon, and still another before retiring.

Hygienic surroundings and an ample supply of fresh air play as important a part in the treatment as the food supply. The good results obtained at the various sanitariums are largely due to the fact that these important considerations have not been overlooked.

At Rutland, Massachusetts, where many patients have derived much benefit, the open-air treatment is used, and all alcoholic stimulants are withheld unless especially ordered by the physician. It must be mentioned, however, that only such patients are admitted as are suffering from the first stages of the disease.

The patients are warmly clad both night and day. During the day most of the time is spent out of doors, and some patients even sleep out of doors, and when not out of doors in a cold room constantly supplied with fresh air. Hoods, mittens, and moccasins are necessary as a protection in such an out-of-door life, and blankets are supplied almost without number.

Patients are allowed a warm room for the cold-water baths, which are recommended, and also for dressing, after which time the heat is turned off, not to be turned on again until time to heat the rooms for undressing.

Under this treatment a weekly gain of weight always is looked for, and patients are weighed at regular intervals that the increase may be recorded. The exercise is limited, to assist in accomplishing this gain, while the food supply is greatly in excess of that furnished for a person in health.

Many physicians are wont to send patients to the far West (Colorado or California), and while some have derived benefit from the change, alas, the greater number have been too wasted by the disease to receive permanent good.

Consumption being an infectious disease, it is never wise to have a large number of cases in a single colony. Where large numbers have flocked to localities where the disease has been unknown, the cases have so multiplied that the error of the plan has been made apparent.

## DIET IN SPECIAL DISEASES.

Many patients who make a change of climate (selecting a spot where the elevation is high and the air dry) during the early stages of the disease, are so benefited as to be able to return without suffering materially from the change; while others find it necessary to remain for the rest of their lives, except, perhaps, for short vacation trips.

Specialists of phthisis are agreed in believing that the most gratifying results come from

1. A treatment of the disease in its first stages.
2. A high and dry climate.
3. A liberal supply of fresh cold air.
4. Daily morning cold-water baths (when possible).
5. Light physical exercise in moderation.
6. A liberal supply of easily digested food, known as the stuffing process.

Fats, in the form of cream, butter, olive oil, bacon, and fat of beef, are most important in the dietary of the consumptive, their caloric value being great in proportion to their bulk.

Among proteid foods, eggs play a very important part, as they are acceptable when raw, or may be cooked in a great variety of ways, either alone or in combination with other food materials. Many physicians advise giving a large number of eggs, and cases are recorded where a patient has taken eighteen in a day, beginning with three, and adding one egg each day until this maximum is reached. While patients have gained on such a diet, there are some objections to its use. Patients usually tire of eggs when taken in such large numbers; then, again, being less completely digested than when taken in small numbers, the use of a cathartic is imperative.

Among meats beef holds first place, principally due to the fact that patients tire of it less quickly. The fat of beef is more easily digested than the fat of mutton, which among meats holds second place. Lamb, chicken, poultry, and game, all are introduced into the diet.

Milk may be taken at the close of a meal, or between meals with a biscuit. There are few foods which need be excluded in feeding phthisis patients. It is a fact to be remembered, however, that when an excess of fat is taken the supply of carbohydrates should be diminished.

When digestion becomes impaired by the stuffing process, oftentimes the use of some alcoholic stimulant will be found of great help as an aid to better digestion.

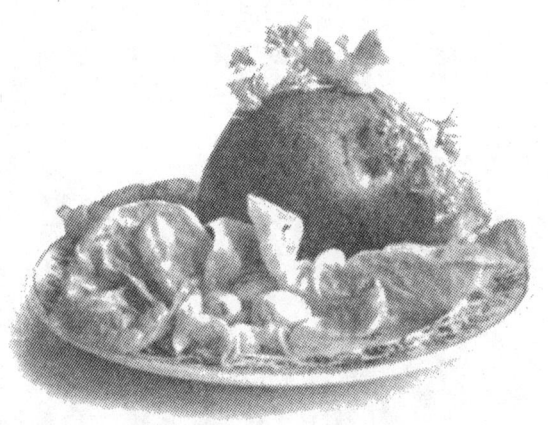

CANARY SALAD
See p. 242

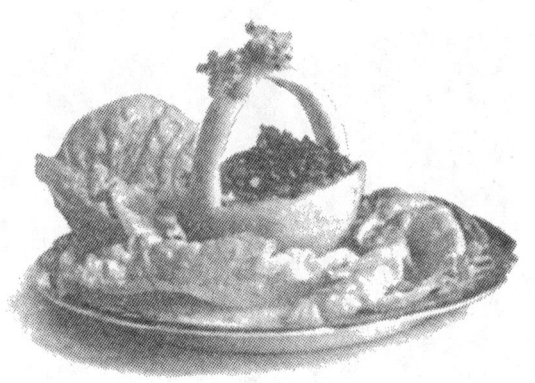

HARVARD SALAD
See p. 242

# INDEX,

## TECHNICAL AND DESCRIPTIVE.

ABSORPTION, defined, 12; 16, 17.
Acid Fermentation, 12.
Acids, 2, 4, 52, 218.
—— Fatty, 16.
Air, essential to life, 1.
Albumen, 2, 44, 52, 108, 217, 259, 260,
Albuminoids, 2.
Albumoses, 13.
Alcohol, 4; absorbed in the stomach, 17; how obtained, 58; a food, 58; avoided by armies and athletes, 58; high proof, 58; absolute, 58; its use in the sick-room, 59; physiological effects of, 59; in diabetic cases, 220.
Alcoholic Beverages, list of, 58; effects produced by, 59; effects produced by habitual use of, 59; conditions which justify use of, 60.
Alcoholic Poisoning, use of coffee in cases of, 65.
Ale, 58.
Alimentary Canal, the, 12; rice water soothing to, 62.
Alkaline Fluids, 12, 16.
Alkaline Reaction, 25.
Alkaloid Thein, 63.
Americans, eat more than other people, 3.
Amides, 2.
Ammonia, 2.
Amylopsin, 16.
Animal Proteids (see Proteids, Animal).
Animals, experiments on, 20.
Anti-toxins, valuable discovery of, 18.
Apollinaris Water, 49.
Apoplexy, 59.

Appetite, the, 1; has marked effect on gastric digestion, 15; best means of stimulating, 37.
Apple, the, calorie value of, 9; time required for digesting, 16; composition of, 203.
Apricots, composition of, 203.
Arabia, 50, 65.
Arrowroot, time required for digesting, 16.
Asia, 50.
Asparagus, composition of, 151, 152.
Asses' Milk, 26.
Assimilation, defined, 12.
Atwater, Prof. W. O., his classification of foods, 2; experiments of, 20; his comparative table showing amount of food required, 34; his table showing composition of fish allowed for the convalescent; 126; his table showing composition of meats used for, 134; his table showing composition of vegetables, 151.

BABY, the, importance of its feeding, 21; requirements of, 21; amount of sleep necessary for, 21; average weight of, 21; earliest feeding of, 22; amount of water required by, 22; importance of regular feeding of, 23; table for feeding, 23; stomach capacity of, 24; a mother's duty to, 24; length of time for each feeding, 26; when best to wean, 30.
Bacon, calorie value of, 9; 39; digestibility of, 139.

# INDEX, TECHNICAL AND DESCRIPTIVE.

Bacteria, 12; not killed by drugs, 13; 26, 46.
Baking, 44.
Baking Powder, 88.
Banana, the, calorie value of, 9; composition of, 203.
Barley, 89.
Barley Gruel, acts as an astringent, 82.
Barley Water, laxative value of, 62.
Bathing, 19; its relation to health, 48.
Beans, 2; time required for digesting, 16.
—— Lima (see Lima Beans).
—— String (see String Beans).
Beat, how to, 43.
Bedouins, the, of Arabia, 50.
Beef, time required for digesting, 15, 16; how to cut it for making beef tea, 84; composition of, 134; nutritive value of, 136; description of a side of, 137; how to determine good, 137; comparative composition before and after cooking, 140.
Beef Extract, Liebig's, calorie value of, 9.
Beef Extracts, described, 83; nutritive value of, 83; how to serve, 84.
Beef Juice, calorie value of, 9.
Beefsteak, calorie value of, 9.
Beef Tea, described, 83; how to use it to advantage, 83; home-made, 83-84.
Beer, 58.
Beet Sugar, 3.
Bermuda Onions, 152.
Beverages, defined, 62; possess little nutritive value, 62; exceptions, 62; what allowed in diabetic diet, 220.
—— Alcoholic, 58.
—— Fruit, 62.
Bile, the, 16; its flow constant, 16.
Bile Pigments, 17.
Bile Salts, the, 16; absorption of, 17.
Biliousness, to prevent, 57; caused by coffee-drinking, 66.
Black Tea, compared with green tea, 63.

Blood, the, dextrose in, 4.
Body, the, relation of food to, 1; food builds and repairs, 1; food furnishes heat and energy for the activities of, 1; principal elements of, 1; quantity of water required by, 5; water constitutes two-thirds the weight of, 5; comparison between locomotive and, 7; the liver acts as storehouse for, 17; uses of water in, 48; vegetables necessary to the needs of, 151.
Body Weight (see Weight, Body).
Boiled Water, 47.
Boiling, 43.
Bomb Calorimeter, the, determines latent energy in different foods, 7.
Bones, the, 5,
Bowels, the, 218.
Brandy (Cognac), calorie value of, 9; 58, 60.
Brazil, 65.
Bread, latent heat in, 7; calorie value of, 9; its effect upon the flow of gastric juice, 14; time required for digesting, 15; the "staff of life," 88; fermented, 88; unfermented, 88; necessary ingredients for a loaf of, 88; what flour best adapted to make, 89; fuel value of, 90; baking of, 93; digestibility of, 93.
—— Entire Wheat, calorie value of, 9.
Bread Dough, 91, 92; shaping, 92.
Bread Making, described, 91.
Breads, Diabetic, 221.
Breakfast Cereals (see Cereals).
Bright's Disease, described, 259; dietetic treatment of, 259-260; foods and condiments not allowed, 260; a day's ration, 261.
Broiling, 43.
Butter, 4; calorie value of, 9; assists digestibility of bread, 93.
Buttermilk, how obtained, 53; its composition, 53; its taste, 53; acts as a laxative, 53.

CAFFEIN, effect of, 65, 67, 83.
Calcium, 52.
Calcium Phosphate, 5.

## INDEX, TECHNICAL AND DESCRIPTIVE.

Calf's Brains, digestibility of, 138.
California, 262.
Calorie, the, defined, 8; table showing number required under different conditions, 10.
Calorie Value, of some important foods, table showing, 9.
Calorimeter, the Bomb, 7.
—— the Respiration, 7.
Cane Sugar, 3, 4; nutritive value of, 4.
Carbohydrates, the, 2; chief office of, 3; include the cheapest kinds of food, 3, 4; waste products of, 4; amount of energy yielded by, 4; 16, 17, 35; aids in the digestion of, 60; 106; the chief source of heat and energy in the body, 218.
Carbon dioxide, 4, 88, 90, 91,
Casein, 2, 52, 55.
Caseinogen, 25, 26.
Cauliflower, time required for digesting, 15; composition of, 151, 152.
Celery, composition of, 151, 153.
Cellulose, 2, 17.
Central America, 65.
Centrifugal Cream, 52.
Cereals, 2, 3, 24, 30, 31; various kinds, 100; valuable, inexpensive foods, 100; table showing composition of, 100; how to obtain best results in cooking, 101; digestibility, 101; table for cooking, 102.
Ceylon, 63.
Champagne, 58, 60.
Cheese, 2; calorie value of, 9; for the diabetic, 219.
Chicken, calorie value of, 9; time required for digesting, 16; digestibility of, 140.
Child, the, birthright of, 21; weaning of, 30; when to feed, 30; what to feed, 31, 32; what not to feed, 32; his craving for sweets, 32; importance of a resting time for, 33; his food at school, 33; why he requires more food to his weight than a man, 34; table showing this comparative amount, 34; table showing increase of calories required for a growing, 35; tea should not be given to, 64. (See also Baby, the.)
Child feeding, viii, 30-35; importance of milk in, 50. (See also Infant feeding.)
Children, require more proteid than the adult, 3; diet of, 5; more readily succumb to disease than older people, 19.
China, 63.
Chittenden, Prof. R. H., experiments of, 20.
Chlorides, 52.
Chlorine, 52.
Chocolate, nutritive value of, 62; manufacture of, 66; gathering of the fruit, 66; composition of, 67; its food value, 67.
—— Sweet, 67.
—— Vanilla, a most desirable food, 32; when injurious, 32, 66.
Cholera, 52.
Cider, 58.
Clam Water, valuable in cases of nausea, 63.
Clams (out of shell), composition of, 126.
Climate, its effect upon foods required, 10.
Cocoa, Breakfast, calorie value of, 9; 24; nutritive value of, 62; manufacture of, 66; gathering of the fruit, 66; composition of, 67; stimulating effect of, 67; its food value, 67.
Cod (salt, boneless), composition of, 126.
Coffee, 1, 24; described, 64; curing of, 64; different grades of, 65; mixtures of, 65; stimulating effect of, 65; how to buy, 65; how to prepare, 65, has no food value in itself, 65; useful in cases of nausea, and opium and alcoholic poisoning, 65, results of excessive drinking of, 66; substitutes for, 66.
—— Java, 65.
—— Mocha, 65.
Cognac, 58.
Colic, 25, 205.

## INDEX, TECHNICAL AND DESCRIPTIVE.

Collagen, of skin and tendons, 2; 134.
Colorado, 262.
Combustion, 1; heat of, 8; process of, 20.
Condiments, 1; allowed in diabetic diet, 220; not allowed in diet for Bright's Disease, 260.
Constipation, 25; usual cause of, 246; effect of diet upon, 246.
Consumption, dietetic treatment of, 261–262.
Contraction, Peristaltic Muscular, 17.
Convalescents, the, tables showing composition of fish allowed for, 126.
Cookery, defined, 41; more attention being paid to subject of, 42; should form part of every woman's education, 42; how to obtain best results in, 42; plays very important part in digestion of foods, 246.
Cooking, Good, importance of, 15, 18.
Corn, Green, 152,
Corn Meal, calorie value of, 10; 89; composition of, 150; how to cook, 102.
Corn Starch, calorie value of, 10.
Cows, most satisfactory breeds of, 27.
Cow's Milk (see Milk, Cow's).
Cracker Gruel, acts as an astringent, 82.
Crackers, Boston, calorie value of, 9.
—— Graham, calorie value of, 9; time required for digesting, 15.
Cranberries, composition of, 203.
Cream, 4; calorie value of, 9; an expensive form of fat, 52; for the diabetic, 219.
—— Centrifugal, 52.
—— Gravity, 52.
Cream of Tartar, 88.
Cream Soups, food value of, 118.
Creams, chemistry of freezing, 197; how to freeze, 197.
Creatin, 83.
Creatinin, 83.
Cucumbers, 152.
Currants, 62.
Cut, how to, 43.

Dates, high food value of, 34; composition of, 203.
Depression, Mental, 67.
Desserts, Frozen (see Frozen Desserts).
Dextrose (see also Grape Sugar), 4, 16.
Diabetes, 60; defined, 217; three stages of, 217; essentially a dietetic disease, 217; in childhood, 217; in adults, 217; diet for, 217–222; necessity of the open air, 222; frequent feeding desirable for, 222.
Diabetes mellitus, 217.
Diabetic Breads, 221.
Diabetic Diet, a, essentials of, 218; proteids in, 218; fats in, 219; vegetables allowed in, 219; fruits, 220; condiments, 220; alcohol, 220; beverages, 220; in detail, 222.
Diabetic Flours, table showing composition of, 221.
Diabetic Milk, Williamson's, 222.
Diarrhœa, 25, 36, 57, 60, 205; defined, 247; diet in cases of, 247.
Diet, importance of, vii; in various diseases, viii; result of abuse of, 11; what kind necessary to preserve normal condition, 14; disease largely due to errors in, 19; average, 217; in diabetes, 218; proteids in, 218; in cases of constipation, 246; in diarrhœa, 247; in indigestion, 248; in hyper-acidity of the stomach, 248; in ulcer of the stomach, 250; in gastritis, 250; in dilated stomach, 251; a fattening, 253; for obesity, 255; for typhoid fever, 257; for rheumatism, 258; for Bright's Disease, 259; for consumption, 261.
"Dietary Computer," the, Mrs. Ellen H. Richards', 11.
Digestion, defined, 12; cases of impaired, 15; principally takes place in the small intestine, 16; temperature of food has marked influence upon, 38.
Digestive Habits, danger of becoming addicted to, 14.

# INDEX, TECHNICAL AND DESCRIPTIVE. 269

Dilation of the Stomach, cause of, 251; treatment of, 252; diet for 250; suggested menu in case of, 252.
Diphtheria, 52, 60.
Disaccharids, 3.
Disease, largely due to errors in diet, 19; important part played by personal idiosyncrasies in, 37; often due to improper feeding, 41.
Diseases, Infectious, due to bacterial action, 18.
Distilled Liquors, 58.
Distilled Water, 46.
Dough, Bread (see Bread Dough).
Dried Fruits, nutritive value of, 204.
Drugs, used less than ever before, 18; do not kill bacteria, 18.
Duodenum, the, 14.
Dysentery, 36.
Dyspepsia, caused by coffee-drinking, 66.

Educators, 30.
Eels, nutritive value of, 125.
Egg-nogs, nutritive value of, 62, 63.
Eggs, Hen's, 2; calorie value of, 9, time required for digestion of, 15; 24; a useful substitute for meat, 106; nutritive value of, 106; composition of, 106; their value in the sick-room, 107; how preserved, 107; how to determine freshness of, 107; advantages of use in sick-room, 108; effects of cooking, 108; digestibility of, 109.
Energy, furnished by food, 1, 7; by proteids, 2, 4; by fats, 4; by carbohydrates, 218.
England, errors of diet in, 19, 20.
Entire Wheat Flour, calorie value of, 9, 10; composition and food value of, 89.
Environment, 19.
Erysipelas, 60.
Evaporated Milk, 82.
Exercise, 19.
Extractives, Meat, 2, 135, 136.
—— Vegetable, 2.

Fæces, 17.
Fat, 25, 217, 218.
Fatigue, produced by tea-drinking, 64.
Fats, 2; furnish heat and energy, 4; amount of energy yielded by, 4, 10, 16; in diabetic diet, 219.
Ferments, 12, 14, 16.
Figs, high food value of, 34; composition of, 203.
Filters, a delusion and a snare, 46.
Fish, 2, 24; described, 125; classification of, 125; nutritive constituents of, 125; not a "brain food," 125; digestibility of, 127.
—— Salt (see Salt Fish).
—— Scaly (see Scaly Fish).
—— Shell (see Shell Fish).
—— White, time required for digesting, 16.
Flavoring extracts, 1.
Flint, experiments of, 20.
Flounder, composition of, 126.
Flour, calorie value of, 9, 10; best kinds for making bread, 89; how to determine strength of, 89; composition and food value of, 89.
—— Entire Wheat, 89.
Flours, Diebetic (see Diabetic Flours).
—— Gluten, 221.
—— Graham, 89.
—— Rye, 89.
—— Wheat, 89.
Fold, how to, 43.
Food, "the only source of human power to work or to think," vii; its relation to the body, 1; builds and repairs the body, 1; furnishes heat and energy for its activities, 1; must undergo changes before utilized by the body, 12; for the baby, 21–29; for the child, 30–35; for the sick, 36–40; must be assimilated to be of value, 37; "well cooked is partially digested," 41; objects in cooking, 41; now stand on a scientific basis, 42.
Food adjuncts, 1; examples of, 1.
Foods, classification of, 2; fuel values of, 7; table showing calorie value

## INDEX, TECHNICAL AND DESCRIPTIVE.

of some important, 9; digestibility of, 15, 16; importance of the study of, 18; their effect on metabolism, 19.

—— Animal, 2; in a diabetic diet, 218.

—— Proteid, chemical elements found in, 2; most expensive, 3.

—— Vegetable, 2; abound in starch, 44, in a diabetic diet, 218.

Fortified Liquors, defined, 58.

Fould's Wheat Germ, how to cook, 102.

Fowl, digestibility of, 140.

Freezer, an Ice-Cream, improvised, 196.

Frozen Desserts, in the sick-room, 196; high food value of, 196

Fruit, 24; chief value of, 35; composition of, 203; possess little food value, 203; nutritive value of, 204, cooking of, 204; digestibility of, 204; danger in eating unripe, 205; what allowed in diabetic diet, 220; in cases of constipation, 247.

Fruit Beverages, 62.

Fruit Sugar, 3, 204.

Fruits, Dried (see Dried Fruits).

Fusel-oil, 59.

GAME, time required for digesting, 16.

Gastric Digestion, 13; influence of extremes in temperature on, 14; Pawlow's experiments, 14; appetite has marked effect on, 15; effect of alcohol upon, 59.

Gastric Disorders, 4.

Gastric Juice, 6, 13, 14, 16; each food calls forth a special, 50; 248.

Gastritis, treatment of, 250; diet for, 250.

Gelatin, 13.

Gelatinoids, 2.

Germany, sanitariums and hospitals in, 15.

Germs, enter system in different ways, 18.

Gin, 58.

Glands, the, 12.

Globulin, 52.

Glucoses, 3.

Gluten, 2, 89.

Gluten Flour, 221.

Glycerine, 16.

Glycogen, 17.

Graham Flour, 89; composition and food value of, 89, 90.

Grape Sugar, 3, 217.

Grapes, 62; composition of, 203.

Gravity Cream, 52.

Green Corn, 152.

Green Tea, compared with black tea, 63.

Gruel, Barley (see Barley Gruel).

—— Cracker (see Cracker Gruel).

—— Thickened Milk (see Thickened Milk Gruel).

Gruels, 36; described, 82; how to prepare, 82; nutritive value of, 82.

HADDOCK, composition of, 126.

Halibut, calorie value of, 9; composition of, 126.

Ham, digestibility of, 139.

Hard Water, 47.

Harrington, Dr. Charles, his table showing composition of diabetic flours, 221.

Headache, produced by tea-drinking, 64.

Health, defined, 18; necessary conditions for, 18; relation of bathing to, 48.

Heartburn, caused by coffee-drinking, 66.

Heart Trouble, 256.

Heat, furnished by food, 1, 7; by proteids, 2, 4; by fats, 4; its application for boiling or steaming, 43, 44; furnished by carbohydrates, 218.

Herrings, nutritive value, 125.

Holmes, Dr. Oliver Wendell, quoted, 18.

Hominy, calorie value of, 10; 31; composition of, 100, how to cook, 102.

Honey, 3.

Hospitals, in Germany, 15; classification of dietaries in, 39, 40.

# INDEX, TECHNICAL AND DESCRIPTIVE. 271

Hot Sulphur Spring Water, 49.
Human Milk (see Mother's Milk).
Hunyadi Water, 49.
Hutchison, 35.
Hyper-acidity, of the stomach, 248; diet suggested for, 240.

ICE-CREAM Freezer (see Freezer, an Ice-Cream).
Ices, chemistry of freezing, 197; how to freeze, 197.
Impaired Digestion, cases of, 15.
India, 63.
Indian Meal, nutritive value of, 82.
Indigestion, causes of, 248; remedies suggested for, 248.
Infant, the (see Baby, the).
Infant feeding, vii., 4, 21–29; table for, 23.
Infectious Diseases, due to bacterial action, 18.
Ingredients, ways of combining, 43.
Insomnia, produced by tea-drinking, 64; by coffee-drinking, 66.
Intemperance, distilled liquors largely responsible for, 58.
Intestine, the large, 17; the small, 14, 16, 17.
Invert Sugar, 3.
Invertin, 16.
Iron, 552.
Italy, 20, 101.

JAPAN, 20, 63.
Java Coffee, 65.
Jessen, 141.
Johannis Water, 49.
Johnston, 140.

KEFIR, composition of, 53.
Kidney Trouble, 72.
Kidneys, the, 259.
König, 25, 140.
Koumiss, manufacture of, 53; its value in the sick-room, 53; home-made, 54.

LACTALBUMIN, 25, 26.
Lactose (see also Milk Sugar), an expensive fuel food, 52.
Lævulose (see also Fruit Sugar), 16.

Lamb Chop, calorie value of, 9; time required for digesting, 16.
Lamb, nutritive value of, 138; how to determine good, 139
Languor, caused by coffee-drinking, 66.
Legumen, 2.
Lemons, 62; composition of, 203.
Lentils, 2.
Lettuce, composition of, 151, 153.
Liebig, on metabolism, 20.
Liebig's Beef Extract, calorie value of, 9.
Life, air essential to, 1; nitrogen essential to, 2; can be sustained on proteids, mineral matter, and water, 3.
Lima Beans (green), composition of, 151.
Lime, Phosphate of, 5.
Lime Water, 26.
Liquors, Distilled, very largely responsible for intemperance, 58.
Lithia Water, 49.
Liver, the, 16; acts as storehouse for the body, 17; fatty degeneration of, 59.
—— composition of, 219.
Lobsters, composition of, 126.
Locomotive, the, comparison between the body and, 7.
Londonderry Lithia Water, 49.
Lunch Counters, in schools, 34.
Lunches, at school, 33; what to put in, 33; what to leave out, 34.
Lungs, the, 4.

MACARONI, composition of, 100, 101, 154.
Mackerel, Spanish, composition of, 126.
Magnesium, 5, 52.
Maleberry Java Coffee, 65.
Mal-nutrition, results of, 19, 248.
Malt Extracts, 60.
Malt Sugar, 3.
Malted Foods, 60.
Maltose (see Malt Sugar).
Man, calories required by, 10; experiments upon, 20.

## INDEX, TECHNICAL AND DESCRIPTIVE.

Maple Sugar, 3.
Mare's Milk, 26, 53.
Massachusetts, legal standard of milk in, 54.
Mastication, necessity of thorough, 12.
Matzoon, composition of, 53.
Meal, Corn, calorie value of, 10.
Measures and Weights, table of, 42.
Meat, 2; latent heat in, 7; its effect upon the flow of gastric juice, 14; 24, 25; described, 134; table showing composition of, 134; structure of, 135; nutritive value of, 135; effects of cooking, 140; losses in cooking, 140; digestibility of, 141.
Meat Extractives, 135, 136.
Mental Depression, due to tea-drinking, 64.
Metabolism, 1, 3, 8; waste products of, 17; effects of foods upon, 19; defined, 19; investigation of, 20; goes on rapidly where temperature is high, 36; effect of alcohol upon, 59.
Mexico, 65, 66.
Milk, Asses' (see Asses' Milk).
—— Cow's, calorie value of, 9; its effect upon the flow of gastric juice, 14; time required for digestion of, 15; 24; composition of, 25, 51; compared with human milk, 25, 26; needs to be modified, 26; best adapted for artificial infant-feeding, 26; better from the herd than from single animal, 27; home-modification of, 27; how to syphon, 28; formula for modifying, 28; how to pasteurize, 29; how to sterilize, 29; 30, 31; an ideal food, 50; a food rather than a beverage, 50; how contaminated, 51; pathogenic germs in, 52; the proteid of, 52; ways of preserving, 54; adulteration of, 54; legal standard in Massachusetts of, 54; effects of cooking, 55; digestibility of, 55; its value in the sick-room, 55; advantages of, 56; disadvantages of, 56; adapting it for the sick, 56; altering taste of, 56; improving digestibility of, 57; predigesting, 57; in bread making, 89.
—— Evaporated, 82.
—— Mare's (see Mare's Milk).
—— Mother's (see Mother's Milk).
—— Skim, 52.
—— Sugar, 3; 4; nutritive value of. 4; cost of, 4; 25.
—— Williamson's Diabetic, 222.
Milk Diet, a, objections to, 56; in cases of typhoid fever, 257; 258; in Bright's Disease, 259.
Mineral Matter, 2, 3; necessary for the building of tissues, 5; 25.
Mineral Waters, 49.
Mocha Coffee, 65.
Modification, of milk, 26; at home, 27; formula for, 28.
Monosaccharids, 3, 4.
Mother, the, importance of regular feeding to, 23; her duty to her child, 24; diet of, 24; when best to wean, 30.
Mother's Milk, 22; methods of regulating, 24, 25; the proteid and fat in, 24, 25; composition of, 25; compared with cow's milk, 25, 26.
Mucin, the, 12.
Muscular Contraction, Peristaltic, 17.
Muskmelons, composition of, 203.
Mussels, 118.
Mutton, composition of, 134; nutritive value of, 138; how to determine good, 139.
Myosin, 2.

Naunyn, on Diabetes, 217.
Nausea, 57; toast water valuable in cases of, 62; use of clam water in cases of, 63; use of coffee in case of, 65; 205.
Nitrogen, essential to life, 2; to determine amount in a given food, 8; the excretion of, 8.
Norway, 50.
Nurse, the, her duty in serving food

# INDEX, TECHNICAL AND DESCRIPTIVE.

to the sick, 38; should be a student of the classification of foods, etc., 39.
Nuts, high food value of, 34.

OATMEAL 31; nutritive value of, 82.
Oats, 89.
—— Rolled (see Rolled Oats).
Obesity, cause of, 255; treatment of, 252; diet for, 255–256.
Œsophagus, the, 13.
Oils, the, furnish heat and energy, 4.
Olive Oil, 4; calorie value of, 9.
Onions, composition of, 151, 152.
—— Bermuda, 152.
—— Spanish, 152.
Opium Poisoning, use of coffee in cases of, 65.
Orange Juice, calorie value of, 9.
Oranges, calorie value of, 9; 62; composition of, 203.
Ossein, of bones, 2.
Oven tests, 44.
—— thermometers, 44.
Oxidation, 1.
Oxides, 52.
Oxygen, discovery of, 20.
Oyster Liquor, 69.
Oysters, calorie value of, 9; time required for digesting, 15; composition of, 126.

PALPITATION, of the Heart, caused by coffee-drinking, 66.
Pancreatic Juice, the, 16; its flow suspended except during digestion, 16; contains four ferments, 16.
Pancreatin, Fairchild's, 57.
Pasteurization, of milk, 26, 29.
Pastry, 24.
Patent Medicines, questionable value of, 61.
Pawlow, Prof. J. P., experiments of, on meat extractions, 135.
Peach, calorie value of, 9.
Peas, 2; time required for digesting, 16.
—— Green, composition of, 151.
Pepsin, 13, 14, 16.
Pepsin Powder, 57.
**Peptones (proteids), 4, 13, 52.**

Perch (white), composition of, 126.
Peristaltic Action, 13.
Peristaltic Muscular Contraction, 17.
Pettenkofer, experiments of, 20.
Pettijohn, how to cook, 102.
Phosphorus, 52.
Phosphoric Acid, 135.
Phthisis (see Consumption).
Pineapples, 62; composition of, 203.
Plums, composition of, 203.
Pneumonia, 60.
Poisoning, opium, 65; alcoholic, 65.
Poland Water, 49.
Poor, the, insufficient quantity of proteids used among, 3; tea drinking among, 64.
Pork, composition of, 134; digestibility of, 139.
Porter, 58.
Potash, 135.
Potassium, 5, 52.
Potatoes, 3; calorie value of, 9; time required for digesting, 15; composition of, 151, 159; described, 159; digestibility of, 159; how to serve, 159; baking and boiling, 159, 160.
—— New, not desirable for sick-room, 160.
Poultry, composition of, 134; digestibility of, 139, 140.
Priestley, discovers oxygen, 20.
Proteids, chief office of, 28; waste products of, 2; give intense heat, 4; 13, 16; absorbed in the stomach, 17; 25, 106, 135, 136, 218; in diet, 218.
—— Animal, 2.
—— Vegetable, 2.
Protein, 2.
Prunes, Dry, calorie value of, 9; composition of, 203.
Ptyalin, defined, 12.

QUAILS, digestibility of, 140.

RASPBERRIES, 62; composition of, 203.
Rectum, the, 17.
Rectal Feeding, 250.
Red Wine, 58, 60.

Rennin, 13, 50.
Respiration Calorimeter, the, 7.
Rest, 19.
Restlessness, caused by coffee drinking, 66.
Rheumatism, dietetic treatment of, 258.
Rice, calorie value of, 9, 10; composition of, 100, 101; how to cook, 102; 154
Rice Water, soothing to the alimentary canal, 62.
Rich, the, tendency to an excess of proteids among, 3.
Richards, Mrs. Ellen H., her "Dietary Computer," 11.
Roasting, 43, 45.
Rolled Oats, calorie value of, 9; composition of, 100; how to cook, 102.
Rolled Rye Flakes, how to cook, 102.
Rum, 58.
Rusks, time required for digestion of, 15; 30.
Russia, 20, 53.
Rutland, Mass., open-air treatment of consumption at, 262.
Rye Flour, 89; composition and food value of, 89.

SACCHARINE, 221.
Sago, 3.
Sago Gruel, time required for digesting, 16.
Sahara, the, 50.
Salad Greens, 153; have little food value, 163.
Salads, described, 163.
Saliva, defined, 12.
Salmon, nutritive value of, 125; composition of, 126.
Salt, 6.
Salt Fish, less digestible than fresh fish, 128.
Salt Pork, digestibility of, 139.
Salts, 13; absorbed in the stomach, 17.
—— the Bile, 16.
Sandwiches, requisites for preparation of, 168.
**Sanitariums**, in Germany, 15.

Saratoga Water, 49.
Scaly Fish, 125.
Scarlet Fever, 52.
Schools, food of a child at, 33; lunch counters at, 34.
Schroeder, 35.
Seltzer, 49.
Service, for the sick, 38; directions for, 38.
Shad, composition of, 126.
Shell Fish, 125.
Sherry, calorie value of, 9.
Sherry Wine, 58, 61.
Sick, the food for, 36–40; their feeding a question of supreme moment, 36; should not be consulted regarding menu, 36; should rarely be awakened for feeding, 36; important things to consider in feeding, 37; appetite of, 37; how to serve food for, 37, 38; methods employed for cooking for, 41; adapting milk for, 56; eggs for, 107, 108; table showing composition of meats used for, 134.
Skim Milk, 52.
Skin, the, 4.
Sleep, 19.
Smelts, composition of, 126.
Soap, 16.
Soda, 88.
Soda Water, 49; assists gastric digestion, 49.
Sodium, 5, 52.
Sodium Chloride, 6.
Soft Water, 47, 48.
Soup-making, 45, 118, 141.
Soup Stock, 118.
Soups, divided into two great classes, 118.
South America, 66.
Spanish Onions, 152
Spices, 1.
Spinach, composition of, 151, 152.
Sponge, a, described, 92.
Squabs, digestibility of, 140.
Squash, composition of, 151, 152.
Starch, digestion of, 13.
—— Animal (see Glycogen).
Starches, 2, 3; examples of, 3, 4;

# INDEX, TECHNICAL AND DESCRIPTIVE.

compared with sugars, 4; 16, 39; vegetable foods abound in, 44, 154.
Steaming, 43.
Steapsin, 16.
Sterilization, of milk, 26, 29.
Stews, the making of, 45.
Stir, how to, 43.
Stomach, the, sugar absorbed by, 4; 12; cut showing division of, 13; has two muscular movements, 14; capable of great distention, 14; plays small part in digestion, 16; vegetables throw much mechanical work on, 154; troubles of, 248; hyper-acidity of, 248; ulcer of, 250; dilation of, 251.
Stomach Trouble (see Indigestion).
Stout, 58.
Strawberries, calorie value of, 9; 62; composition of, 203.
String Beans (green), composition of, 151.
Sucrose (see Cane Sugar).
Sucroses, 3.
Sugar, 3, classification of, 3; found in the blood, 4; absorbed in the stomach, 4, 11; a desirable quick-fuel food, 4; compared with starch, 4; calorie value of, 9; 13, 17; does not injure the teeth, 35; completely absorbed by the system, 39; 218; substitutes for, 221.
Sugar Substitutes, 221.
Sulphur, 52.
Sunlight, 19.
Sustoff, 221.
Sweden, 20, 50.
Sweet Chocolate, 67.
Sweetbreads, time required for digesting, 15; described, 138; digestibility of, 138.
Switzerland, 50.

TAMARINDS, 62.
Tannic Acid, 60, 63.
Tannin, 63.
Tapioca, 3; calorie value of, 10; time required for digesting, 16.
Taste, the, all eating much influenced by, 38.

Tea, 1, 24, described, 63; the best brands, 63; differences in quality, a stimulant rather than a nutrient, 63; how to prepare, 63; its food value, 64; evil effects of, 64; a useful stimulant, 64, should never be given to children, 64.
—— Beef (see Beef Tea).
—— Black, 63.
—— Green, 63.
Tea Drinkers, require less food, 64; apt to become nervous, 64.
Teeth, the, 5.
Temperature, influence on gastric digestion of, 14.
Thein, effect of, 63, 65, 67, 83.
Theobromine, 67.
Thermometers, Oven, 44.
Thickened Milk Gruel, acts as an astringent, 82.
Thompson, Sir Henry, on errors of diet, 19.
Tissue, Connective, 17.
Tissues, built and repaired by proteids, 2.
Toast Water, valuable in cases of nausea, 62.
Toasted Wheat, how to cook, 102.
Tomatoes, composition of, 151, 152.
—— Canned, calorie value of, 9.
Tremor, caused by coffee drinking, 66.
Trout, composition of, 126.
Trypsin, 16.
Tuberculosis, 52.
Turbot, composition of, 126.
Typhoid Fever, 52; causes of, 257; diet for, 257; frequent feeding desirable in, 258.

ULCER of the stomach, 250; treatment of, 250; diet for, 250.
U. S. Department of Agriculture, bulletins of, 8, 100, 106.
Urea, 2.
Urine, the, 2, 4, 217, 222.

VAN NOORDEN, his work on metabolism, 20; 136, 255, 259.
Veal, described, 138.

# INDEX, TECHNICAL AND DESCRIPTIVE.

Vegetable Proteids (see Proteids, Vegetable).
Vegetables, cellulose in, 2; 24; chief value of, 35; table showing composition of, 151; nutritive value of, 151; necessary for the body's requirements, 151; cooking of, 153; digestibility of, 154; throw mechanical work on the stomach, 154; what allowed in diabetic diet, 219.
Vichy, 49.
Vitos, how to cook, 102.
Voigt, experiments of, 20.
Vomiting, 25, 250.

WATER, 2, 3, 4; quantity required by the body, 5; constitutes two-thirds of the weight of the body, 5, 46; 13; amount required by a baby, 22; 25, 30, 37; amount required by an adult, 46; component parts of, 46; not chemically pure in nature, 46; source of derivation for household consumption, 47; the greatest known solvent, 47; temperatures of, 47; uses in the body, 48; has many uses of valuable importance to man 48; a valuable antiseptic, 49; Nature's beverage, 62.
—— Boiled, 47.
—— Distilled, 46; chemically pure, 46.
—— Hard, described, 47; can be rendered soft. 48.

Water, Soft, 47, 48.
—— Well, location should be carefully examined, 47.
Water Cures, 49.
Water Temperatures, 47.
Weaning, a child, 30.
Weight, Body, how to increase, 253.
Weights and Measures, table of, 42.
Well Water, 47.
West Indies, the, 66.
Wheat Breakfast Cereal, composition of, 100.
Wheat Flour, 89.
Wheat Germ, calorie value of, 10.
Wheatena, how to cook, 102.
Wheatlet, calorie value of, 10; how to cook, 102.
Whey, 53.
Whiskey, calorie value of, 9, 58.
White Sulphur Spring Water, 49.
White Wine, 58.
Whitefish, composition of, 126.
Williamson's Diabetic Milk, 222.
Wine, Red, 58.
—— White, 58.
Wine Whey, uses of, 62.

YEAST, 53, 88; described, 90; conditions favorable for its growth, 90; in bread making, 90–92.
Yeast Cakes, 91; how to know when fresh, 91.

ZWIEBACK, 30, 92, 168.

# INDEX TO RECIPES.

ALBUMEN,
    Brandy, 225.
    Claret, 225.
    Madeira, 72.
    Orange, 72, 225.
    Port, 72.
    Sherry, 72.
    Water, 68.
        with Beef Extract, 68.
Albumenized Milk, 74.
Almond,
    Cakes, 226.
    Tarts, 195.
Angel Drop Cakes, 212.
Apple,
    Sauce, 205.
        Baked, 206.
        Strained, 205.
    Tapioca Pudding, 173.
    Velvet Cream, 244.
    Water, 68.
Apricot, Dried, Sauce, 206.
    Strained, 207.
Apricot and Wine Jelly, 183.
Asparagus,
    Boiled, 154.
    on Toast, 154.
    Salad, 240.
    Soup, 119, 230.
    Tips, Creamed, 155.
    with Milk Toast, 154.

BACON, Curled, 145.
Banana, 207.
    Baked, 207.
    How to serve, 207.
Barberry Jelly Water, 69.
Barley,
    Gruel I., 85; II., 85.
    Water, 67.
Bavarian Cream, Coffee, 244.

Beans,
    Shell, 155.
    String, 155.
Béchamel Sauce, 150.
    Yellow, 150.
Beef,
    Balls, 141.
    Broiled Steak, 142.
        with Sauce Figaro, 233.
    Broiled Tenderloin with Beef Marrow, 149.
    Jelly, 183.
    Pan Broiled Cakes, 142.
    Roast, with Horseradish Cream Sauce, 234.
    Fillet of, 234.
Beef Extract, 86.
    Frozen, 87.
    with Albumen Water, 68.
    with Chicken Soup, 228.
    with Port, 87.
Beef Jelly, 183.
Beef Omelet I., 114; II., 116.
Beef Sandwiches,
    Raw, 169.
    Toasted, 170.
Beef Tea, I., 87; II., 87; III., 87.
Beet Greens, 156.
Beverages, 62–81.
    Albumen, 72, 225.
        Brandy, 225.
        Claret, 225.
        Madeira, 72.
        Orange, 72, 225.
        Port, 72.
        Sherry, 72.
        Water, 68.
             with Beef Extract, 68.
    Chocolate, 62, 66, 81.
    Clam Water, 73.

Beverages (cont.),
  Cocoa, 62, 66, 79, 80.
    Brandy, 80.
    Breakfast I., 80; II., 80.
    Cordial, 81.
    Cracked, 79.
    Shells, 79.
      and Cracked Cocoa, 80.
  Coffee, 64, 76, 78, 79.
    Black, 79.
    Cereal, 79
    Filtered, 78.
    Pot of, 78.
    with Butter, 223.
    with Cream, 223.
    with Egg, 223.
  Egg-Nog I., 76; II., 76; 225.
    Coffee, 76.
    Cream, 225.
    Fruit, 225.
    Hot Water, 76.
    Pineapple, 76.
  Egg with Brandy, 77.
  Flaxseed Tea, 72.
  Fruit, 62, 68-72.
    Apple Water, 68.
    Barberry Jelly Water, 69.
    Crab-apple Jelly Water, 69.
    Currant Jelly Water I., 69; II., 69.
    Grape Juice, 69.
    Lemon Whey, 72.
    Lemonade, 70.
      Egg, 70; I., 224; II., 224.
      with Lactose, 71.
      Flaxseed, 71.
      Hot, 70.
      Irish Moss, 71.
      Soda or Apollinaris, 70.
      with Lactose, 70
    Orange Albumen, 72
    Orangeade, 72, 224.
    Raspberry Shrub, 69.
    Syrup for, 69.
  Ginger Tea, 75.
  Milk, 73-75.
    Albumenized, 74
    Ginger Ale and, 75.
    Hydrochloric, 74.

Beverages (cont.),
  Milk (cont.),
    Junket Whey, 73.
    Koumiss, 74.
    Lemon Whey. 72.
    Peptonized, (cold Process) 73; (warm Process), 74.
    Punch of, 75.
    Sippets with, 99.
    Thickened, 85.
    Williamson's Diabetic, 223.
    Wine Whey, 73
  Moxie with Egg, 76.
  Oyster Liquor, 73.
  Starchy, 62, 67, 68.
    Barley Water, 67.
    Rice Water, 67.
    Toast Water, 68.
  Tea, 63, 77, 78.
    Cup of, 77.
      made with Tea Ball, 77.
    Iced, 77.
      with Mint, 77.
    Pot of, 78.
    Russian, 77.
  Water, 62.
    Albumen, 68.
    Apple, 68.
    Barberry Jelly, 69.
    Barley, 67.
    Clam, 73.
    Crab-apple Jelly, 69.
    Currant Jelly I., 69; II., 69
    Rice, 67.
    Toast, 68.
    Whey, 72.
    Junket, 73.
    Lemon, 72.
    Wine, 73.
Birds, How to bone, 148.
Bisque,
  Mock, 119.
  Tomato, 230.
Blanc Mange,
  Chocolate, 187.
  Irish Moss, 187.
Boning, of Birds, 148.
Bran Muffins, 96.
Brandy,
  Albumen, 225.

# INDEX TO RECIPES. 279

Brandy (cont.),
  Cocoa, 80.
  Sauce, 177.
  with egg, 77.
Bread, 88–99.
  and Butter Pudding I., 172; II., 172.
  and Butter Sandwiches, 169.
  Croustades of, 99.
  Croûtons, 124.
  Entire Wheat I., 94; II., 94.
  Graham, 95.
  Health Food, 96.
  Imperial Sticks, 124.
  Milk and Water, 94.
  Oat, 95.
  Omelet, 115.
  Pudding, Chocolate, 172.
  Pulled, 94.
  Rye, 95.
  Sticks, 96.
  Water, 93.
Broth,
  Chicken, 123.
    with Cream, 123.
    with Egg, 123.
  Mutton, 122.
Brussels Sprouts,
  in White Sauce, 155.
  with Curry Sauce, 235.
Butter,
  Drawn, 149.
  Maître d'Hôtel, 150.
  Sauce, Drawn, 128.
  with Coffee, 223.
Buttered Egg, 226.

CABBAGE Salad, 238.
  and Celery, 238.
Cake, White Corn Meal, 97.
Cakes,
  Almond, 226.
  and Wafers, 211.
  Angel Drop, 212.
  Cream, 214.
  Gluten Nut, 226.
  Lady Fingers, 212.
  Little Sponge, 213.
  Macaroons, Cereal, 215.
  Marguerites, 215.

Cakes (cont.),
  Meringues or Kisses, 216.
  Plain, 214.
  Sponge, 214.
    Little, 213.
    Baskets, 213.
Canary Salad, 242.
Cantaloup Melon, How to serve, 210
Caramel,
  Ice Cream, 200.
  Junket, 190.
  Custard, 188.
    Baked, 189.
    Steamed, 188.
Cauliflower,
  à la Huntington, 235.
  Creamed, 155.
  Fried, 235
  Soup, 120, 230.
  with Hollandaise Sauce, 235.
Celery,
  and Sweetbread Salad, 168.
  Curled, 156.
  with Cheese, 236.
Celeried Oysters, 133.
Charlotte Russe, 194.
  Caramel, 194.
  Chocolate, 194.
  Coffee, 195.
  Strawberry, 195.
Cheese,
  Balls, 237.
  Custard, 237.
  Rarebit, 237.
  Salad, 167, 239.
    and Egg, 239.
    and Olive, 239.
    and Tomato, 240.
  Sandwiches, 237.
  with Celery, 236.
  with Halibut, 232.
Chicken,
  and Nut Salad, 243.
  and Rice Cutlets, 147.
  Broiled, 145.
  Broth, 123.
    with Cream, 123.
    with Egg, 123.
  Creamed, 146.
  Jelly, 184.

## INDEX TO RECIPES.

Chicken (cont.),
    Maryland, 146.
    Purée, 123.
    Roast, 146.
    Salad, 168.
    Sandwiches, 170.
        Chopped, 171.
    Soufflé, 147.
    Soup,
        with Beef Extract, 228.
        with Egg Balls, 229.
        with Egg Custard, 228.
        with Royal Custard, 229.
    Suprême of, 236.
    Timbale of, 147.
Chocolate, 62, 66, 81.
    Bread Pudding, 172.
    Corn Starch Pudding, 174.
    Cottage Pudding, 175.
    Custard, Steamed, 188.
    Frozen, with Whipped Cream, 201.
    Ice Cream, 200.
    Irish Moss Blanc Mange, 187.
Chops,
    Broiled Lamb, 142.
    Pan Broiled French, 143.
Christmas Jelly, 184.
Cider Jelly, 183.
Clam,
    Soup, 122.
    Water, 73.
Clams, 127.
Claret Albumen, 225.
Cocoa, 62, 66, 79, 80.
    Brandy, 80.
    Breakfast I., 80; II., 80.
        with Egg, 80.
    Cracked, 79.
    Shells, 79.
        and Cracked Cocoa, 80.
    with Tapioca, 191.
Coddled Egg, 112.
Codfish,
    Creamed, 131.
    Salt, 127.
        with Cheese, 233.
        with Cream, 233.
Coffee, 64, 76, 78, 79.
    Bavarian Cream, 244.

Coffee (cont.),
    Black, 79.
    Cereal, 79.
    Custard,
        Baked, 190.
        Steamed, 188.
    Egg-Nog, 76.
    Filtered, 78.
    Ice Cream, 200.
    Jelly, 183.
    Pot of (boiled), 78.
    with Butter, 223.
    with Cream, 223.
    with Egg, 223.
    with Tapioca, 191.
Cold Desserts, 187–195.
Cole Slaw, 238.
Concord Ice Cream, 201.
Cookies, Scotch, 211.
Corn Meal,
    Cake, White, 97.
    Mush, 103.
    Pudding, 175.
Corn Starch Pudding, 174.
Cottage Pudding, 174.
Crab-Apple Jelly Water, 69.
Cracker,
    Gruel, 84.
        Dextrinized, 84.
    Toast, 98.
Crackers, Crisp, 124.
Cranberry,
    Jelly, 207.
    Sauce, 207.
Cream,
    Apple Velvet, 244.
    Cakes, 214.
    Cocoa, 193.
    Coffee Bavarian, 244.
    Dressing I., 164; II., 164
    Egg-Nog, 225.
    Filling, 215.
    Hamburg, 192.
    Horseradish, 234.
    of Celery Soup, 120.
    of Corn Soup, 120.
    of Pea Soup, 119.
    Orange, 192.
    Sauce, with Smelts, 233.
    Sherbet, Lemon, 245.

# INDEX TO RECIPES.

Cream (cont.),
    Spanish, 193.
        Coffee, 193.
    Toast, 99.
    Wine, 192.
    with Coffee, 223.
Creamed
    Cauliflower, 155.
    Chicken, 146.
    Fish, 130.
    Oysters, 133.
    Peas, 157.
    Potatoes, 161.
    Sweetbread, 144.
Creamy Sauce I., 176; II., 177.
Crisps, Wheat, 211.
Croustades of Peas, 157.
Croûtons, 124.
Cucumber,
    and Egg Salad, 239.
    and Leek Salad, 238.
    and Sweetbread, 243.
    and Water-cress Salad, 238.
    Boats, 243.
    Cup, 238.
    Sauce, 231.
Currant Jelly Water I., 69; II., 69.
Curry Sauce, with Brussels Sprouts, 235.
Custard,
    Baked, 189.
        Caramel, 189.
        Cheese, 237.
        Coffee, 190.
        French baked, 195.
        Purity, 189.
        Royal, 229.
    Junket, 190.
    Junket, Caramel, 190.
    Soufflé, 175.
    Steamed, 187.
        Caramel, 188.
        Chocolate, 188.
        Coffee, 188.
DANDELIONS, 156.
Dextrinized Cracker Gruel, 84.
Diabetic, the recipes for, 223–255.
Diabetic Milk, Williamson's, 223.
Dip Toast, 99.
Drawn Butter Sauce, 128, 150.

Dressing,
    Boiled, 164.
    Cream, I., 164; II., 164.
    French, 164.
    Mayonnaise, 165.
    Oil, 165.
Dried Apricot Sauce, 206.
    Strained, 207.
Drinks (see Beverages).
Drop Cakes, Angel, 212.
Dry Toast, 98.
Duchess Potato, 161.

EGG,
    à la Suisse, 227.
    Baked, 111.
        in Tomato, 228.
    Balls, I., 229; II., 229.
        with Chicken Soup, 229.
    Buttered, 226.
    Coddled, 112.
    Custard with Chicken Soup, 228
    Dropped I., 110; II., 111.
        with Tomato Purée, 227.
        with White Sauce, 111.
    Farci I , 227; II., 227.
    "Hard Boiled," 110.
    in Nest, 112.
    Lemonade, 70.
        I. 224; II., 224.
        with Lactose, 71.
    Omelets, 114–117.
    Salad I., 166, 239; II., 167, 239
        and Cheese, 239.
        and Cucumber, 239.
    Sandwiches, I., 170; II., 170.
    Sauce, 129.
        I., 149; II., 149.
    Scrambled I., 111; II., 112.
    Shirred, 111.
    "Soft Boiled," I., 110; II., 11 .
    Soufflé, 113.
    Souffled, 112.
    Steamed, 228.
    Timbale, 113.
    with Brandy, 77.
    with Breakfast Cocoa, 80.
    with Coffee, 223.
    with Moxie, 76.
    with Wheat Mush, 103.

## INDEX TO RECIPES.

Egg-Nog,
  I., 75; II., 75.
  Coffee, 76.
  Cream, 225.
  Fruit, 225.
  Hot Water, 76.
  Pineapple, 76.
Eggs,
  à la Buckingham, 113.
  a la Goldenrod, 113.
  au Beurre Noir, 226.
Entire Wheat, 94.
  Bread I., 94; II., 94.
  Sandwiches, 169.

Farina Gruel, 85.
Fever, Recipe for Cases of, 75.
Fig Sandwiches, 171.
Figaro Sauce, 233.
  with Broiled Beefsteak, 233.
Figs, Stewed, 207.
Fillet of Haddock, 232.
Filling, Cream, 215.
Fineste Sauce, 234.
  with Lamb Chops, 234.
Finnan Haddie, à la Delmonico, 232.
Fish,
  Clams, 127.
  Creamed, 130.
  Finnan Haddie, 232.
    à la Delmonico, 232.
  Haddock, 232.
    Baked, 232.
    Boiled, 129.
    Fillet of, 232.
  Halibut, 232.
    Baked, 232.
    Fillet of, 130, 231.
      Baked, 130.
    Steamed, 128.
    Timbale, 130.
    with Cheese, 232.
  Lobster, 127.
  Oysters, 127.
  Salad I., 240; II., 240.
  Salt Codfish, 127, 233.
    Creamed, 131.
    with Cream, 233.
    with Cheese, 233.

Fish (cont.),
  Sardine Relish, 237.
  Smelts, 233.
    a la Maître d'Hôtel, 233.
    with Cream Sauce, 233.
Flaxseed,
  Lemonade, 71.
  Tea, 72.
French Dressing, 164.
Fricassee of Oyster, 132.
Frozen Beef Extract, 87.
  Chocolate with Whipped Cream 201.
  Punch, 245.
  Tomato Salad, 241.
Fruit Beverages,
  Currant Jelly I., 69; II., 69.
  Egg-Nog, 225.
  Grape Juice, 69.
  Lemonade, 70.
  Orange Albumen, 72, 225.
  Orangeade, 72, 224.
  Raspberry Shrub, 69.
  Syrup for, 69.
Fruit Salad I., 210; II., 210.
Fruit Soufflé, 176.
Fruit Sauce, 178.
Fruit (cooked) Sauces,
  Apple, 205.
    Baked, 206.
    Strained, 205.
  Apricot, Dried, 206.
    Strained, 207.
Fruits, Cooked, 203–210.
  Apple, 205.
    Baked, 205.
    Sauce, 205.
      Baked, 206.
      Strained, 205.
    in Bloom, 206.
    Snow, 206.
  Bananas, 207.
    Baked, 207.
  Cranberry, 207.
    Jelly, 207.
    Sauce, 207.
  Figs, 207.
    Stewed, 207.
  Orange, 209.
    Marmalade, 209.

INDEX TO RECIPES. 283

Fruits (cont.),
    Pears, 209.
        Baked, 209.
    Prunes, 209.
        Stewed, 209.

GASTRIC Trouble, Recipes for Cases of, 75.
Ginger Ale, with Milk, 75.
Ginger Tea, 75.
Gingerbread, Hot Water, 212.
Gluten Nut Cakes, 226.
Graham Bread, 95.
Grape Fruit, How to serve, 208.
Grape Fruit Ice, 198.
Grape Juice, 69.
Grape Sherbet, 199.
Grapes, How to serve, 208.
Gruel,
    Barley I., 85; II., 85.
    Cracker, 84.
    Dextrinized Cracker, 84.
    Farina, 85.
    Indian Meal, 86.
    Oatmeal I., 86; II., 86.
    Rice, 84.
    Thickened Milk, 85.

HADDOCK,
    Baked, 232.
    Boiled, 129.
    Fillet of, 232.
Halibut,
    Baked, 232.
    Fillet of, 130, 231.
        Baked, 130, 232.
    Steamed, 128.
    Timbale, 130.
    with Cheese, 232.
Ham,
    Broiled I., 144; II., 145.
Hamburg Cream, 192.
Harvard Salad, 242.
Health Food Bread, 96.
Hollandaise Sauce,
    with Baked Fillet of Halibut, 231.
    with Cauliflower, 235.
Hominy Mush, 103.

Horseradish Cream Sauce, with Roast Beef, 234.
Hot Water Egg-Nog, 76.
Hydrochloric Milk, 74.

ICE Cream, 196–202.
    Caramel, 200.
    Chocolate, 200.
    Coffee, 200.
    Concord, 201.
    Flowering, 201.
    Frozen Chocolate with Whipped Cream, 201.
    in a Box, 201.
    Macaroon, 200.
    Pistachio, 200.
    Vanilla, 199.
Iced Tea, 77.
    with Mint, 77.
Ices, 198, 199.
    Cup St. Jacques, 201.
    Grape Fruit, 198, 245.
    Lemon, 198.
    Orange, 198, 245.
    Pineapple, 198.
    Raspberry, 199.
    Strawberry, 199.
Imperial Sticks, 124.
Indian Meal Gruel, 86.
Invalid Muffins, 97.
Irish Moss,
    Blanc Mange, 187.
    Chocolate, 187.
    Fruit Blanc Mange, 186.
    Jelly, 71.
    Lemonade, 71.

JELLY Omelet, 116.
Jelly Sandwiches, 171.
Jelly, 71, 103, 179–184.
    Apricot and Wine, 183.
    Beef, 183.
    Chicken, 184.
    Christmas, 184.
    Cider, 183.
    Coffee, 183.
    Cranberry, 207.
    Irish Moss, 71.
    Ivory I., 180; II., 180.
    Lemon I., 180; II., 180.

Jelly (cont.),
    Macedoine Pudding, 186.
    Oat, 103.
    Orange, 180.
        in Surprise, 185.
        Sauce, 175, 185.
        with sections of Orange, 181.
    Orange Baskets with, 181.
    Pears in, 186.
    Port I., 182; II., 182.
    Rice, 179.
    Sauterne, 184.
    Stimulating, 182.
    Tapioca I., 179; II., 179.
    Veal, 184.
    Wine I., 181; II., 182.
Junket,
    Caramel, 190.
    Custard, 190.
    Whey, 73.

KISSES or Meringues, 216.
Koumiss, 74.

LACTOSE,
    with Egg Lemonade, 71.
    with Lemonade, 70.
Lady Fingers, 212.
Lamb Chops,
    Broiled, 142.
        with Sauce Fineste, 234.
    Pan Broiled French, 143.
Leek and Cucumber Salad, 238.
Lemon,
    Cream Sherbet, 245.
    Ice, 198.
    Jelly I., 180; II., 180.
    Sauce, 177.
    Soufflé, 176.
    Whey, 72.
Lemonade, 70.
    Apollinaris, 70.
    Egg, 70; I., 224; II., 224.
        with Lactose, 71.
    Flaxseed 71.
    Hot, 70.
    Irish Moss, 71.
    Soda, 70.
    with Lactose, 70.

Lettuce, 156.
    Dressed, 166.
    Sandwiches, 170.
Lobster, 127.

MACARONI,
    Baked, 105.
    Boiled, 104.
    with Oysters, 105.
    with White Sauce, 104.
Macaroon Ice Cream, 200.
Macaroons, Cereal, 215.
Macedoine Pudding, 186.
Madeira Albumen, 72.
Maître d'Hôtel Butter, 150.
Marguerites, 215.
Marmalade, Orange, 209.
Mayonnaise Dressing, 165.
Meat, ways of cooking, 141.
    Beef, 141.
        Balls, 141.
        Cakes, Pan Broiled, 142.
    Beefsteak, Broiled, 142.
    Lamb, 142.
        Broiled Chops, 142.
        Pan Broiled French Chops 143.
    Pork, 144.
        Bacon, 145.
            Curled, 145.
        Broiled Ham I., 144; II. 145.
    Soufflé, 236.
    Sweetbread, 143.
        Creamed, 144.
        Glazed, 144.
        Jellied, 144.
Meringues or Kisses, 216.
Milk,
    Albumenized, 74.
    Ginger Ale and, 75.
    Hydrochloric, 74.
    Koumiss, 74.
    Peptonized (cold Process), 73.
        (warm Process), 74.
    Sippets with, 99.
    Thickened, 85.
    Williamson's Diabetic, 223.
Milk Punch, 75.
Milk Sherbet, 199.

Milk Toast, 98.
    with Asparagus, 154.
Mint Cup, Orange, 210.
Moxie with Egg, 76.
Muffins,
    Bran, 96.
    Invalid, 97.
Mush,
    Corn Meal, 103.
    Hominy, 103.
    Rolled Oats, 102.
    Wheat, with Egg, 103.
    Wheatlet, with Fruit, 102.
Mushroom Soup, 230.
Mushrooms,
    Broiled, 236.
    in Cream, 236.
Mutton Broth, 122.

Nut and Chicken Salad, 243.
Nut Cakes, Gluten, 226.

Oat,
    Bread, 95.
    Jelly, 103.
    Wafers, 211.
Oatmeal Gruel, I., 86; II., 86.
Omelet, 114–117.
    Beef I., 114; II., 116.
    Bread, 115.
    Cereal, 116.
    Foamy I., 114; II., 114.
    French, 116.
    Jelly, 116.
    Orange, 116.
    Oyster, 115.
    with Peas, 115.
Onions, Boiled, 156.
Orange,
    Albumen, 72, 225.
    Baskets,
        with Jelly, 181.
    Cream, 192.
    Ice, 198, 245.
    in Surprise, 185.
    Jelly, 180.
        with sections of Orange, 181.
    Marmalade, 209.
    Omelet, 116.

Orange (cont.),
    Puffs, 175.
    Sauce, 175, 185.
    Ways of serving, 208.
Orangeade, 72, 224.
Oyster,
    Liquor, 73.
    Omelet, 115.
    Soup, 121.
    Stew, 121.
Oysters,
    Baked in Shells, 131.
    Broiled, 133.
    Celeried, 133.
    Color of, 127.
    Creamed, 133.
    Fancy Roast, 132.
    Fricassee of, 132.
    Grilled, 132.
    How to wash, 132.
    Omelet of, 115.
    Raw, 131.
        with Sherry, 131.
    Season of, 127.
    Stewed, 121.
    with Macaroni, 105.

Peach Snow, 210.
Peach Tapioca Pudding, 173.
Pears, Baked, 209.
Peas,
    Creamed, 157.
    Croustades of, 157.
    Green, 157.
    in Tomato Basket, 167.
    Omelet with, 115.
Peptonized Milk,
    (cold Process), 73.
    (warm Process), 74.
Pineapple Egg-Nog, 76.
    Ice, 198.
Pistachio Ice Cream, 200.
Pork, 144.
    Bacon, Curled, 145.
    Ham, Broiled, I., 144; II., 145.
Port Albumen, 72.
    Jelly, I., 182; II., 182.
    with Beef Extract, 87.
Potato Soup, I., 118; II., 119.

Potatoes, 159.
    au Gratin, 162.
    Baked, 160.
    Balls I., 162; II., 162.
    Boiled, 160.
    Border, 162.
    Creamed, 161.
    Duchess, 161.
    Mashed, 161.
    Riced, 161.
    Served in Shell, 160.
    Steamed, 161.
    Ways of Cooking, 160–162.
Princess Pudding, 244.
Prune Souffle, 192.
Prunes, Stewed, 209.
Puddings,
    Baked,
        Apple, 173.
        Cream of Rice, 173.
    Bread and Butter, I., 172; II., 172.
    Chocolate,
        Bread, 172.
        Corn Starch, 174.
        Cottage, 175.
    Corn, 175.
    Cottage, 174.
        Chocolate, 175.
    French, 245.
    Hot, 172–176.
    Marshmallow Pudding, **186**.
    Orange Puffs, 175.
    Princess, 244.
    Snow, I., 185; II., 185.
    Soufflé,
        Custard, 175.
        Fruit, 176.
        Lemon, 176.
    Tapioca,
        Apple, 173.
        Custard, 174.
        Peach, 173.
Punch, Frozen, 245.
Purée, Chicken, 123.
Purity Custard, Baked, 189.
QUAIL, Broiled, on Toast, 147.
RADISHES, Ways of Cutting, 166.
Rarebit for the Diabetic, **237**.
Raspberry Ice, 199;
    Shrub, 69.

Relish, Sardine, **237**.
Rice,
    Boiled, 103.
    Gruel, 84.
    Jelly, 179.
    Steamed, 104.
    Water, 67.
Riced Potatoes, 161.
Rolled Oats Mush, 102.
Royal Custard, 229.
Rusks (Zwieback), 97.
Russian Tea, 77.

SALAD, 163, 166–168.
    Asparagus, 240.
    Cabbage, 238.
        and Celery, 238.
        Cole Slaw, 238.
    Canary, 242.
    Cheese, 167, 239.
        and Olive, 239.
        and Tomato, 240.
    Chicken, 168.
        and Nut, 243.
    Cucumber Cup, 238.
        and Egg, 239.
        and Leek, 238.
        and Sweetbread, 243.
        and Water-cress, 238.
        Boats, 243.
    Dressed Lettuce, 166.
    Egg I., 166, 239; II., 167, 239
        and Cheese, 239.
        and Cucumber, 239.
    Fish I., 240, II., 240.
    Fruit I., Sweet, without dressing, 210: II., 210.
    Harvard, 242.
    Nut and Chicken, 243.
    Spinach, 243.
    Sweetbread, 168.
        and Cucumber, 243.
    Tomato I., 167; II., 167, **241**.
        and Chive, 242.
        Basket of Plenty, 241.
        Basket with Peas, 167.
        Frozen, 241.
        Jelly, 241.
            with Vegetables, **241**.
        **Stuffed, 242.**

## INDEX TO RECIPES.

Salad Dressings, 163-165.
  Boiled, 164.
  Cream I., 164; II., 164.
  French, 164.
  Mayonnaise, 165.
  Oil, 165.
Sandwiches, 168-171.
  Beef, 169.
    Raw, 169.
    Toasted, 170.
  Bread and Butter, 169.
  Cheese, 237.
  Chicken, 170.
    Chopped, 171.
  Egg I., 170; II., 170.
  Entire Wheat, 169.
  Fig, 171.
  Jelly, 171.
  Lettuce, 170.
  Sweet, 171.
Sardine Relish, 237.
Sauce, Fruit, 178.
Sauces of cooked fruit,
  Apple, 205.
    Baked, 206.
    Steamed, 205.
  Apricot, Dried, 206.
    Strained, 207.
Sauces, for
  Meat and Fish, 149, 150.
    Béchamel, 150.
      Yellow, 150.
    Cream, 233.
    Cucumber, 231.
    Drawn Butter, 128, 149.
    Egg Sauce I., 149; II., 149.
    Figaro, 233.
    Fineste, 234.
    Hollandaise, 231.
    Horseradish Cream, 234.
    Maître d'Hôtel, 150, 233.
    Tomato, 150, 232.
    White Sauce II., 149.
    White Wine, 232.
  Puddings, 175-178.
    Brandy, 177.
    Cream I., 176; II., 177.
    Fruit, 178.
    Hard, 176.

Sauces, for (cont.),
  Puddings (cont.),
    Lemon, 177.
    Orange, 175.
    Whipped Cream, 177.
    Wine, 177.
  Vegetables, 149.
    Curry, 235.
    White Sauce I., 149.
Sauterne Jelly, 184.
Scalloped Fish, 130.
Scotch Cookies, 211.
Scottish Fancies, 212.
Serve, How to,
  Bananas, 207.
  Cantaloup Melon, 210.
  Grape Fruit, 208.
  Grapes, 208.
  Oranges, 208.
Sherbet,
  Grape, 199.
  Lemon Cream, 245.
  Milk, 199.
Sherry Albumen, 72.
Shrub, Raspberry, 69.
Sippets with milk, 99.
Slaw, Cole, 238.
Smelts,
  à la Maître d'Hôtel, 233.
  with Cream Sauce, 233.
Snow Pudding I., 185; II., 185.
Soufflé of Meat, 236.
Souffléd Egg, 112.
Soup,
  Accompaniments, 124.
  Asparagus, 119, 230.
  Cauliflower, 120, 230.
  Chicken,
    with Beef Extract, 228.
    with Egg Balls I., 229; II., 229
    with Egg Custard, 228.
    with Royal Custard, 229.
  Clam, 122.
  Cream of Celery, 120.
  Cream of Corn, 120.
  Cream of Pea, 119.
  Mock Bisque, 119.
  Mushroom, 230.
  Onion, 229.
  Oyster, 121.

Soup (cont.),
    Potato I., 118; II., 119.
    Spinach Soup, 120, 231.
    Tomato, 121.
        Bisque, 230.
    Triplex, 122.
Spinach,
    Boiled, 157, 234.
    Salad, 243.
    Soup, 120, 231.
Sponge,
    Cakes, 214.
    Baskets, 213.
    Little, 213.
Squab, Boned, in Paper Case, 148.
Squash, Winter, Steamed, 158.
Strawberries, 209.
Strawberry Ice, 199.
String Beans, 155.
Suprême of Chicken, 236.
Sweetbread,
    and Celery Salad, 168.
    and Cucumber Salad, 243.
Sweetbreads,
    Broiled, 143.
    Creamed, 144.
    Glazed, 144.
    Jellied, 144.
Syrup, for Fruit Beverages, 69.

TAPIOCA,
    Cream I., 191; II., 191.
    Custard Pudding, 174.
    Jelly I., 179; II., 179.
    Pudding, 173.
        Apple, 173.
        Peach, 173.
    with Cocoa, 191.
    with Coffee, 191.
Tarts, Almond, 195.
Tea, 63, 77, 78.
    Beef, I., 87; II., 87; III., 87.
    Cup of, 77.
        with Tea Ball, 77.
    Flaxseed, 72.
    Ginger, 75.
    Iced, 77.
        with Mint, 77.
    Pot of, 78.
    Russian, 77.

Timbale,
    Chicken, 147.
    Halibut, 130.
Toast,
    Cracker, 98.
    Cream, 99.
    Croustades of Bread, 99.
    Dip, 99.
    Dry, 98.
    Milk, 98.
        with Asparagus, 154.
    Sippets with Milk, 99.
    Water, 68, 98.
Toasted Beef Sandwiches, 170.
Tomato,
    and Chive, 242.
    Basket of Plenty, 241.
        with Peas, 167.
    Bisque, 230.
    Frozen, 241.
    Salad I., 167; II., 167.
    Sauce, 150, 232.
    Soup, 121.
    Stuffed, 242.
    with Baked Halibut, 232.
    with Baked Egg, 228.
Tomatoes,
    Broiled, 158.
    Sliced, 158.
    Stewed, 158.

VANILLA Ice Cream, 199.
Veal Jelly, 184.
Vegetables,
    Asparagus, 154.
        Boiled, 154.
        on Toast, 154.
        Tips, Creamed, 155.
        with Milk Toast, 154.
    Beans, 155.
        Shell, 155.
        String, 155.
    Beet Greens, 156.
    Brussels Sprouts, 155, 235.
        in White Sauce, 155.
        with Curry Sauce, 235
    Cauliflower, 155, 235.
        à la Huntington, 235.
        Creamed, 155.
        Fried, 235.

Vegetables (cont.),
Cauliflower, with Hollandaise Sauce, 253.
Celery, 156, 236.
    Curled, 156.
    with Cheese, 236.
Dandelions, 156.
Lettuce, 156.
Mushrooms, 236.
    Broiled, 236.
    in Cream, 236.
Onions, Boiled, 156.
Peas, 157.
    Creamed, 157
    Croustades of, 157.
    Green, 157.
    in Tomato Basket, 167.
Potatoes, 159.
    au Gratin, 162.
    Baked, 160.
    Balls I., 162; II., 162.
    Boiled, 160.
    Border, 162.
    Creamed, 161.
    Duchess, 161.
    Mashed, 161.
    Riced, 161.
    Served in Shell, 160.
    Steamed, 161.
    Ways of cooking, 160–162.
Sauces for, 149.
Spinach, 157, 234.
    Boiled, 157.
Squash, Winter, Steamed, 158.
Tomatoes, 158.
    Broiled, 158.
    Sliced, 158.
    Stewed, 158.

WAFERS, 211.
    Oat, 211.
Water,
    Albumen, 68.
    Apple, 68.
    Barberry Jelly, 69.
    Barley, 67.
    Clam, 73.
    Crab-apple Jelly, 69.
    Currant Jelly I., 69; II., 69.
    Rice, 67.
    Toast, 68, 98.
Water Bread, 93.
Water-cress and Cucumber Salad, 238.
Water Toast, 98.
Wheat Crisps, 211.
Wheat Mush with Egg, 103.
Wheatena with Fruit, 102.
Wheatlet Mush with Fruit, 102.
Whey,
    Junket, 73.
    Lemon, 72.
    Wine, 73.
Whipped Cream, 177.
White Corn Meal Cake, 97.
White Sauce I. (for Vegetables), 149, II. (for Meat and Fish), 149.
White Wine Sauce, with Fillets of Haddock, 232.
Williamson's Diabetic Milk, 223.
Wine and Apricot Jelly, 183.
Wine Cream, 192
Wine Jelly I., 181; II., 182.
Wine Sauce, 177.
    Whey, 73.
Winter Squash, Steamed, 158.

ZWIEBACK (Rusks), 97.

www.ingramcontent.com/pod-product-compliance
Lightning Source LLC
LaVergne TN
LVHW031629070426
835507LV00024B/3390